"A to Z Book of Natural Hair Loss Solutions"

Author
James M. Merritt, Jr.

FOREWORD

"A to Z Book of Natural Hair Loss Solutions"

JAMES M. MERRITT, JR.
COPYRIGHT 2015

This work is intended for the private use of the purchaser. Contents of this book are suggestive in nature and are no substitute for sound medical advice when required.

DEDICATION

"This work is dedicated to all people who attempt to make this a better world to live in."

ACCESSIBILITY

*Availability of ingredients may vary based upon multiple conditions. In those cases we provide access to similar highest quality substitutes based upon marketplace conditions.

TABLE OF CONTENTS

TABLE OF CONTENTS CONT'D

"A to Z Book of Natural Hair Loss Solutions"

Ladies and Gentlemen you might be simply stunned to find out that literally hundreds of unpublicized ingredients have been tested as cures for baldness. This research has taken place at leading universities and medical centers throughout the world. Some of these products such as Upjohn's Rogaine and Merck's Propecia did find their way to the marketplace but the vast majority garnered little publicity in research. The simple reason for this is that it would take millions of dollars to bring them to the consumer, whether they were approved or not by the United States Food and Drug Administration (FDA). The offshoot of this testing though was that quite a few of these unpublicized compounds did show an astounding ability to either curb hair loss, totally halt it, or promote hair regrowth. To finalize the bottom line if you can't totally regrow a full head of hair unquestionably the next best thing is to halt or prolong your hair loss for as long as possible and obtain as much regrowth as you can. Plus preferably you would like to do this at as cheaply as possible. What's also great about these ingredients is they can be used in conjunction with hair transplants if you choose that route.

INTENTION OF INFORMATION

This compilation is meant to tell you about some of these unique ingredients that many people have found to be astoundingly cheap methods for combating hair loss. By providing this information it is our intention to help individuals establish a program which they can embark upon for retarding hair loss and establishing new hair growth. Plus when we say cheap none of these products should cost you much over five dollars, with the exception of a few. In those cases we'll tell you where to obtain the products at prices considerably below what many companies are charging. Quite a few of our suggestions will also reflect upon various methods of use for these ingredients, to increase their effectiveness and decrease their costs to you.

In regard to program it is important to point out the success or failure of any individual routine can vary significantly. Proper usage is always advised to obtain the best results. Since no product whether a prescription medication or OTC ingredient has ever shown complete effectiveness for hair loss, it is understandable why results would vary widely. Our course is to point out the compounds so you can establish a direction for yourself. We also encourage consulting with a skilled hair stylist to fit a hairstyle to your face and body. This can be highly beneficial since no ingredient has been proven to work overnight. Remember success in any endeavor is dependent on a positive outlook.

We would also like to point out that we do not endorse the products of any one manufacturer over another nor do we represent any manufacturer or sales group. Our views are merely suggestive in nature and may be contrary to many others. We also may change our approval status on various ingredients based upon established effectiveness, safety records, and price declines in the marketplace.

ANALYSIS OF PATTERN BALDNESS

To understand how these ingredients work it is appropriate to give a short discussion on why male and female pattern baldness exhibits itself in certain portions of our population. Assuming the fact that the individual involved is in good health, the reason alopecia occurs seems to be linked to a certain genetic predisposition, which is common in quite a few individuals. This is not to say that poor nutrition, use of various drugs (legal or illegal), thyroid conditions, pregnancy, metabolism, areata, or possibly serious medical conditions among many things don't cause hair loss. It is only to clarify that pattern baldness is predominantly the result of heredity. But that doesn't mean the results of heredity can't be altered. As extensive study has shown pattern baldness can occur among both sexes at many ages. The end result of course being a thinning of the hair on the scalp in varying degrees. As the Norwood Process points out there are seven stages to the thinning process, each with progressively more hair loss.

The scientific reasoning for pattern baldness is that the thinning process is thought to be related to a decrease in circulation, until genetically predisposed hair follicles shut down. According to scientists when it comes time to go bald the hair follicles in the scalp markedly increase the production of testosterone 5-alpha reductase. This enzyme converts testosterone made in other parts of the body to dihydrotesterone (DHT), which in turn makes the hair stop growing. Administration of hormones taken orally or applied topically can reverse hair loss but not without sometimes-serious side effects. Scalp injections of higher quality forms of testosterone with fewer side effects are still being tested today and may one day prove an effective treatment for pattern baldness.

One of the important things that should be pointed out is that cholesterol formation that produces the enzyme testosterone 5-alpha reductase also takes place as the result of sunlight producing it on the skin and scalp. So in theory if you can reduce the amount of this enzyme on the scalp combining with testosterone to create dihydotestosterone (DHT), you could in practice retard hair loss.

As you might guess by now the theory behind some of these ingredients is to disrupt some of this aforementioned activity from occurring on the scalp, increase the circulation, and provide optimal conditions for regrowth. Used properly these ingredients should produce anti-androgen effects that would lessen the resultant hair loss from 5-alpha reductase. They are not miracle potions but relatively cheap solutions that can be used in a weekly regime to obtain the desired results. At worse these ingredients will provide you with a fuller, healthier, and thicker looking head of hair than you've probably ever had before. On the other hand many people have found these products do exactly what they desire, which is to retard hair loss and obtain various degrees of hair regrowth.

We will now tell you about some of these ingredients and what products contain them. By all means the ingredients are not limited to the formulations we are going to tell you about. You should always keep an eye out for even more affordable combinations. Plus for those who have access to pharmaceutical quality or cosmetic solutions that avenue is always possible. Through this process you can greatly understand what hair care products you may be already using on your scalp and how it effects hair growth. If you are a student of history you might find since the days of the Egyptians early herbal remedies dealt with ways to reduce 5-alpha reductase (DHT) on the scalp.

- **As the authors of these works have always maintained pattern baldness has it roots in multiple disciplines. This being the case we offer dozens of alternatives for your consideration.**

- **Researchers at the University of Pennsylvania claim to have made a major breakthrough in the baldness battle by inhibiting a single enzyme, prostaglandin D2 (PGD2),**

which they say is the "major" enzyme connected to hair loss.

SUGGESTIONS FOR USAGE

With all of the suggested ingredients we urge discontinuance if scalp irritation or redness becomes obvious. In the case of pharmaceutical or herbal agents for internal consumption we recommend stoppage if side effects become noticeable or evident. Following the prescribed directions for usage is always advisable. Data on some well-known ingredients for hair loss has not been included in these writings. The reasoning behind this is that safe consumption has not been determined for these agents over extended periods of time. Furthermore most of these products will never be marketed for anything outside of their intended purpose.

One other caution we would especially like to give emphasis to is the overuse of vitamins, herbs, and nutrients. More is not necessarily better. We say this because there is a small percentage of people who "load up" on every vitamin, supplement, and ingredient they can put their "hands on". This is very unwise and can often lead to side effects. We advise testing out a few ingredients at a time, at the suggested dosage. If after one to three months they appear to work for you, continue with them. If not, discontinue and try some others. Just don't abuse it. Mega-dosing usually just creates a drain on your pocketbook.

NATURAL HAIR LOSS INGREDIENTS GROUP A

ALFALFA

Alfalfa is one of those rare ingredients where there is a consensus that it slows hair loss and can prolong the growth phase of the follicle but it has never gained widespread usage for those purposes. One thing is for certain this legume contains an abundance of nutrients crucial to hair growth such as vitamin B2, B5, and folic acid. It also contains trace amounts of copper, zinc, manganese and magnesium. Even though alfalfa has found more usage in Ayruvedic medicine it stills follows the same principles as Chinese practitioners do for halting hair loss. Namely the ingredient promotes better liver function and reduces cholesterol. Cholesterol being one of the building blocks of DHT.

This legume inherits its name from the Arabic word which literally means the "father of all plants". Plus it's easy to see why it gains this notoriety when the root system can extend downward thirty feet or more. By doing so it draws trace minerals into its structure otherwise not found in shallow root plants.

Bottom line alfalfa being a food supplement makes it one of the more natural ways to fight hair loss.

SOURCES FOR ALFALFA

1. **Various Alfalfa Supplements**
   http://www.iherb.com
   http://www.swansonvitamins.com
2. **Rusk Full Green Tea & Alfalfa Shampoo**
   http://www.beautydeals.net
   http://www.diamondbeauty.com
   http://www.thebeautyplace.com
3. **J Beverly Hills Men Thickening Shampoo**
   http://www.fashionandbeautystore.com

ALOE VERA

Aloe Vera the "miracle plant" has a soothing, moisturizing effect on the scalp. It contains salicylates, the identical pain killing substances found in aspirin. This member of the Lilly family also contains magnesium, zinc, all of the B-vitamins, plus biotin, choline, and inositol. Twenty-two amino acids, polysaccharides, and glucose can similarly be added to this list. That's mighty impressive for one ingredient.

The soothing lotion of this plant also has the molecular weight to penetrate skin tissue and dilate the capillaries, thereby increasing the blood supply to the application area. Its moisture retention capabilities are remarkably high. The extracts are one of the better natural cleansing agents for the skin and scalp, because of their anti-bacterial properties.

Dating back to the times of Alexander the Great, Nero, and Discorides aloe has been prescribed as a tonic for hair loss. A possible reason for these claims might dwell upon the fact that aloe has the ability to inhibit the immune response. Some scientists point to the fact that over activity of the immune system may be a determinative factor in hair loss. Many forms of dermatitis react positively to this plant's ingredients. The medicinal qualities are almost too abundant to list for this wondrous herb.

PRODUCTS CONTAINING ALOE VERA

1. **Thicker Fuller Hair Shampoo and Conditioner**
2. **Nexus Hair Care Products**
3. **Vitamin and Nutrition Stores**
4. **GNC Stores Aloe Vera Shampoo**
5. **Biotene H-24 Shampoo and Conditioner**
6. **Tom's of Maine Aloe and Almond Hair Care Products**
7. **Aveda Shampoos and Conditioners**
8. **Focus Sea Plasma Shampoo**
   http://www.haircareusa.com
9. **Jason Natural Aloe Vera Shampoo**
   http://www.drvita.com
   http://www.vitasprings.com/shampoo.html
10. **Mill Creek Aloe Vera Shampoo**
    http://www.iherb.com
    http://www.millcreekusa.com
11. **Chamovera Shampoo and Conditioner**
    http://www.baar.com

ALPHA LIPOIC ACID

Alpha Lipoic Acid also known as thiotic acid is probably one of the most potent antioxidants available in the marketplace today. Derived from red meats it is often used by vegetarians because it is not produced in quantity by the human body. This vitamin like substance seems to derive its highest level of potency when combined with the supplements C and E. Some scientists maintain that "caramelization" is why our bodies are in a continuous state of aging and that subsequently is the reason we lose our hair. Since we are continuously exposed to stress, pollutants, and various stimuli this caramelization process is accelerated in many of us. Hair loss being a major symptom of this acceleration. Even though this antioxidant possesses no qualities that would initiate hair growth anecdotal evidence suggests consuming it retards hair loss substantially.

Europeans who often consume many more natural products, for the prevention of disease than Americans, utilize Alpha Lipoic Acid to the greatest degree. In fact European research has long maintained this ingredient is one of the more effective supplements for treating glaucoma, hair loss, and diabetes.

SOURCES FOR ALPHA LIPOIC ACID

1. **GNC - General Nutrition Stores.**
2. **Health and Nutritional Stores**
3. **Herbs Wholesale**
   http://www.herbs-wholesale.com
4. **American Nutrition**
   http://americannutrition.com
5. **Vitamin Express**
   http://www.vitaminexpress.com
6. **Best Vite**
   http://www.bestvite.com

AMLA

Amla or Indian Gooseberry is one of the many wondrous herbs of India derived from the tree native to that country. Described as one the better sources for vitamin C (ascorbic acid), the herb itself has been linked to many anti-aging properties related to the skin and hair. Consumed orally the herb has been documented to lower cholesterol and increase red blood cell counts.

The active ingredient that has significant pharmacological action is designated as phyllemblin. Other ingredients present are gallic acid, tannins, pectin, amino acids, copper, superoxide dismutase, linolenic acid, and zinc.

For years the extracts of this plant have been used in hair tonics that claim to rejuvenate hair growth and return the pigmentation of the hair to its original state. The reasoning behind this is that the herb may prevent rancid lipid peroxidation of the scalp, increase the anti-inflammatory response, or its cholesterol lowering capabilities may counteract DHT formation. Used as a hair rinse it is purported to be one of the better hair conditioners to be found. Some people have gone as far as to label Amla as a "natural minoxidil" but more research is needed before this euphemism can be properly applied.

SOURCES FOR AMLA

1. **Shikai Natural Hair and Skin Care**
   http://www.ihealthtree.com
   http://www.shikai.com
2. **Shahnaz Herbal**
   http://mall.coimbatore.com/bnh/shahnaz/haircare.h
   tm
3. **Kalyx.com - Hair Oils**
   http://www.kalyx.com
4. **Better Botanicals Shampoo Amla Shine**
   http://www.allvitaminsplus.com
   http://www.supplementwarehouse.com
5. **Neeta's Herbal Amla Shampoo**
   http://www.vitaliving.com

APPLE JUICE

An interesting concept that originated from Japanese research is the use of green apples to halt hair loss. In theory components found within green apples were able to halt hair loss when applied topically. Interestingly enough the research never evolved because comparative studies showed that the same results could be obtained from drinking the juices of this fruit, whether it was green or not.

The reasoning behind the cessation of hair loss and promotion of regrowth was linked to vitamin B-2 (procyanidin). Supposedly the phtyo-chemicals within the fruit decreased swelling in the hair follicle allowing hair growth. Similar to an inflammation or immune response this swelling once reduced allowed the hair follicle to produce at optimal levels. Since aloe and Emu oil seem to work by a similar process of lessening the immune response the remedy is not totally without merit.

As a treatment some people have crushed the juices an applied externally or consumed them internally. The simplest route though is to find a distributor for natural apple juice that contains a high percentage of the natural ingredients. If you have access to a juicer you can make your own.

SOURCES FOR APPLE JUICE

1. **Grocery and Natural Food Stores**
2. **Produce Stands**

APPLE POLYPHENOLS

One of the bigger buzz phrases in the hair loss world is apple polyphenols. Receiving much of its publicity from Japanese research the extracts from this fruit have proven to be potent hair growth agents. Apparently the procyanidins within this fruit, specifically B-2 and C-1, are capable of suppressing PKC in both the anagen (active growth phase) and telogen (resting phase) of the hair follicle thereby leading to hair regrowth in those experiencing pattern baldness. The PKC's being protein kinase C isozymes. What's unique about the extracts is they have been shown to work either by internal consumption or topical application. These apple extracts have also been shown to aid in fat metabolism allowing many to lose weight and gain muscle mass at the same time. Because the extracts are drawn from the skins of the apple, where the sugars are not present, it can be helpful in reversing some diabetic conditions.

SOURCES FOR APPLE POLYPHENOLS

1. **Swanson Vitamins**
   http://www.swansonvitamins.com
2. **Applepoly**
   http://www.applepoly.com

ARGININE

Arginine is one of the essential amino acids. By this we mean the human body cannot create it so it must be obtained from the foods we consume. This amino acid is chiefly found in meats such as chicken and turkey plus dairy products. The nutrient itself has been shown to induce growth hormone release in humans. Normally by the time we reach our early thirties the release of this chemical stimulus has ceased. High intensity exercise though can facilitate the secretion of this hormone.

Proponents of using actual human growth hormone or amino acids such as Arginine and Orthinine argue that it can turn back the aging clock. Their research indicates that the presence of this hormone can rejuvenate many of our physiological functions considerably. In a percentage of people who do react favorably to these particular amino acids, body fat is noticeably reduced and lean muscle mass is increased. Visually detectable increases in skin elasticity and noticeable hair growth were observed in many cases.

If you desire to take these amino acids research indicates that they work best if you lead an active lifestyle. Bottom line these nutrients do boost physical performance and increase hair growth in many instances. These amino acids can also be purchased fairly cheaply in many retail vitamin sections.

SOURCES FOR ARGININE

1. **Arginine is most often found in vitamin and nutrition stores. Typical store formulas will contain both Arginine and Orthinine. Research seems to indicate that these nutrients work best in combination.**
2. **Yves Rocher Hair Care**
    http://www.yvesrocherusa.com
3. **Avalon Organics Peppermint Shampoo**
    http://www.certifiedorganic.org
4. **Redken Intra Force System 1&2**
5. **Redken Climatress**
6. **L'Oreal Paris Arginine Resist X3**
7. **Renokin Hair Revitalizing Shampoo**
    http://hairloss101.com
8. **Redken Extreme Shampoo**
    http://www.drugstore.com
    http://www.usabeautysupplies.com

AROMATHERAPY

Aromatherapy is the usage of various oils to enhance the well-being of the individual. Each of the essential oils has its own character and can be used by itself or blended with other oils to obtain the desired effect. These oils can be used to help a wide variety of ailments both physical and emotional as well as those that are stress related.

For years practitioners of aromatherapy have claimed that the oils were very beneficial in treating hair loss and growing hair. This has largely been anecdotal until a recent British study validated quite a few of these claims. This double blind clinical study concluded that when various essentials oils were employed nearly half of the patients showed marked improvement in their hair loss situations. Eighty-four patients were involved in the study. The oils used were thyme, lavender, rosemary, and cedarwood. The carrier oils utilized were grape seed and jojoba oils. Carrier oils are used to dilute the essential oils for massage into the scalp. Without them many of the essential oils would be far too strong to apply directly to the skin. Typical concentrations are one drop of the essential oil per 5ml of the carrier oil. Clary, sage, and Ylang are some other recommended essential oils for hair loss.

AROMATHERAPY PRODUCTS

1. **Essential and Carrier Oils can be found at select Health and Nutritional Stores or through various holistic and aromatherapy practitioners.**
2. **Samson's Secret**
    http://www.samsonssecret.com
3. **Mountain Rose Herbs**
    http://mountainroseherbs.com
4. **Aromaland Aromatherapy Shampoo**
    http://www.aromaland.com
5. **American Crew Trichology Hair Recovery**
    http://www.haircareusa.com
6. **Stimulate Shampoo**
    http://www.escentsaromatherapy.com

AVOCADO OIL

Avocado oil is one of the few natural botanicals that have a tiny enough molecular mass to be absorbed deeply into the skin and hair follicle. This being so allows it to mimic sebum which keeps the hair shaft soft and subtle while at the same time increasing its flexibility. Based upon this it is no small wonder why this oil is a prized ingredient in many better hair loss and skin care products. Plus it becomes even better because various vitamins found in the avocado are able to piggyback their anti-oxidant and anti-bacterial properties straight into the skin. These being such things as vitamin A,B,C,D,E, plus lecithin which aid in retarding the aging process. Bottom line since it is an oil though its benefits for hair loss likely come from the fatty acids, vitamin E, lutein, the phytosterol content (in particular beta sterol), and carotenoids.

SOURCES FOR AVOCADO OIL

1. **Redken All Soft Shampoo**
2. **Organix Acai Berry Avocado Shampoo**
3. **Peter Lamas Avocado Olive Ultra Smoothing Shampoo**
   http://www.soap.com
4. **Giovanni 2chic Avocado & Olive Oil Ultra-Moist Shampoo**
   http://www.vitaminlife.com

AZELAIC ACID

One ingredient that everybody seems to be making a mad rush for is Azelaic acid. This substance is a naturally occurring saturated dicaroxylic acid extracted from barley, wheat, and rye. It has been around for quite a few years as a treatment for acne and other skin conditions. According to French studies it is a very potent DHT inhibitor and even more potent when combined with zinc and vitamin B-6. Unlike Retonic Acid, which has its greatest value when combined with minoxidil, this acid's benefits can be derived without the latter. Research indicates it is effective on the frontal hairline. Azelaic Acid is manufactured by Schering Pharmaceuticals under the name Skinoren. It is a prescription drug. Used in moderation, on the frontal hair-line, a $22 tube can last about three months.

SOURCES FOR AZELAIC ACID

1. **Doctor's Prescription**
   http://www.4rx.com
   http://www.4cornerspharmacy.com
   http://www.eurodrugstore.eu
2. **Min of New York Secure DHT Inhibitor Styling Gel**
   http://www.onlyhairloss.com
   http://hairlosstoregrowth.com
   http://www.salonweb.com
3. **Revivogen Shampoo**
4. **Wholesale Hair Products**
   http://www.wholesalehairproducts.com
5. **AzaClear OTC product now available in United States.**

NATURAL HAIR LOSS INGREDIENTS GROUP B

BERGAMOT

Bergamot is one of the essential oils with a sweet spicy aroma found in the Rutaceaa genus. The oils are derived from the peel of the fruit of the same name that looks much like a cross between an orange and a lemon. It is in the same family as the orange tree and is harvested mainly in southern Italy from trees that grow to a height of about fifteen feet. The oil itself has an emerald color and the smell and taste can be best understood because it is an ingredient used in Earl Grey Tea.

The Romans used bergamot as a hair growth stimulant among a long list of ingredients to combat hair loss. The oil is now primarily used an antiseptic and soothing agent. It is also used by some of the more expensive hair loss products such as FNS Osmotics as a hair loss preventative and as means to stimulate scalp circulation.

SOURCES FOR BERGAMOT

1. **Rusk Sensories Healthy Blackberry & Bergamot Strengthening Shampoo**
   http://www.salonsavings.com
   http://www.beautycarechoices.com
   http://www.verbenaproducts.com
2. **Bergamot Shampoo and Hair Tonic**
   http://www.bonanza.com
3. **Bergamot Shampoo**
   http://www.thaiherbalproducts.com
4. **Tommy-Guns Bergamot and Inula Shampoo**
   http://www.nivenandjoshua.com

BETA SITOSTEROL

Beta Sitosterol is basically an herbal agent containing a mixture of phytosterols. Its popularity is beginning to grow as a substitute for saw palmetto. It contains far more sterols than the latter. These sterols seem to be highly beneficial in the treatment of prostate troubles and the retardation of hair loss. Beta Sitosterol can also be processed from sugar cane and other plant sources far more cheaply than saw palmetto.

In European tests of the active ingredients of beta sitosterol results indicated it was just as effective as many prescription pharmaceuticals in treating benign prostatic hyperplasia (BPH). The question though still remained, after these tests, as to exactly what mechanism of action enabled Beta Sitosterol to produce its results. Since this has never been established, beta sitosterol has never quite achieved the status many manufacturers would like it to.

Beta Sitosterol normally exhibits its results within a month of usage with regards to hair loss. There should be a noticeable slowing of hair fallout after that. Since this ingredient is naturally derived, with no side effects, it should always be considered an essential in any arsenal to combat hair loss.

SOURCES FOR BETA SITOSTEROL

1. **This supplement can be found at many health and nutritional stores.**
2. **Food Science of Vermont Superior Hair**
   http://www.vitacost.com
   http://www.swansonvitamins.com
   http://www.luckyvitamin.com
3. **I Herb**
   http://www.iherb.com
4. **The Vitamin Shoppe**
   http://www.vitaminshoppe.com
5. **Natrol Beta Sitosterol**
   http://www.thepowerstore.com
6. **Source Naturals Beta Sitosterol**
   http://www.vitacost.com

BHRINGARAJ OIL

Bhringaraj is an herb long known for its hair restoration capabilities. It can be found growing in India and parts of the southwestern United States. The name means "ruler of the hair." Practitioners of Ayruvedic medicine maintain it corrects the khalitya and palitya allowing for proper hair growth, when applied to the scalp. Similar to the Chinese belief that hair loss is related to liver dysfunction, Bhringaraj has long been used as treatment for cirrhosis. Studies have shown the oil itself possesses anti-inflammatory qualities that seemingly enhance hair growth. To use just apply to the areas of the scalp that are thinning.

SOURCES FOR BHRINGARAJ OIL

1. **Ayruvedic Herbs Direct**
   http://www.ayurvedicherbsdirect.com
2. **Auromere Pre-Shampoo Conditioner**
   http://www.ayurvedicbazaar.com
   http://www.iherb.com
3. **Banyan Botanicals - Massage and Herbal Oils**
   http://www.banyanbotanicals.com
   http://www.drugnatural.com

BILBERRY EXTRACT

Bilberry is a plant closely related to blueberries and currants. The most important quality of this unique herbal being the tannins as well as vitamin A and C. The specific activity of Bilberry comes from the concentrated fruit pigments called anthocyanins. These anthocyanins have a strengthening effect upon the blood vessel walls.

In relation to hair loss when utilized in hair lotions or capsule form blood flow is enhanced in the scalp area. Bilberry is able to do this by increasing the collagen within the blood vessel's outer wall to allow for optimal flow of the blood. It also exhibits potent antibacterial and antiviral activity when applied to the skin.

Amazingly the standard application of Bilberry is for the reduction eyestrain and improving night vision. In addition to helping minute capillaries supply blood to the eye, it helps produce the color purple in our visual field. The color purple is essential for helping us convert light into electrical signals for the brain to produce our vision.

The best way to try out Bilberry is in capsule form, if you don't have access to the oils in a hair lotion. Hair loss reduction should become apparent within two weeks if it is going to work for you.

SOURCES FOR BILBERRY EXTRACT

1. **Walmart Stores**
2. **GNC Stores**
3. **Health and Nutritional Stores**

4. **Solgar Bilberry Extract**
5. **Wonder Laboratories**
    http://www.wonderlabs.com
6. **Whole Health**
    http://www.wholehealth.com

BIMATOPROST

Oddly enough the hottest hair loss ingredient to be found is an FDA sanctioned ophthalmic treatment from Allergen. It was initially approved as a topically applied drug (Lumigan) to reduce ocular hypertension present in glaucoma. It later found approval from the same agency as a cosmetic eyelash growth agent (Latisse) for the treatment of hypotrichosis (lack of eyelashes). The active ingredient of both formulas being Bimatoprost.

The story started when purchasers of the product begin to experiment with the eyelash formula on the frontal hairline. Much to their surprise small vellus hairs along the hairline began to darken, thicken, and lengthen. As this information spread a few California dermatologists begin testing and prescribing it to a select clientele of Hollywood actors. Based upon the limited conclusions available Bimatoprost is a capable hair restoration agent that produces results often in less than a month if it is going to work for you. Plus the effects tend to be permanent even with discontinuance of the medication. The biggest caveats tend to be a lack of any long term research and the costs. Even though the medication is considered very safe rare occurrences of blue eye pupils growing darker have occurred with glaucoma patients. Among users of Latisse, for the eyelashes, there have been no reported instances of the eye color changing.

It is important to point out that scalp and eyelash hair have similar cycles of loss and renewal. The caveat though is scalp hair is hormone sensitive (DHT) whereas eyelash hair is prostaglandin sensitive (Bimatoprost). Never less some early research indicates this unique compound may insulate the scalp treated hair from the effects of DHT.

*   **There are online pharmacies selling generic Bimatoprost for as little as five dollars a bottle if you can find them. In some cases the quantities are larger than is normally found in a typical container because it has been recognized as a hair growth agent. Quite a large grey**

market as developed as the result of this.

- **Be sure to purchase the 0.3% strength for the best results on your frontal hairline. Coverage of larger areas especially the crown is generally not recommended purely based upon the costs.**

- **Compounding pharmacies offer Bimatoprost in quantity, at greatly reduced prices, if you have access to them.**

<u>SOURCES FOR BIMATOPROST</u>

1. **Pharmacies selling generic Bimatoprost.**
   http://ipharmacylist.com
   http://www.planetdrugsdirect.com
   http://www.canadadrugsonline.com
   http://www.northdrugstore.com

<u>BIOTIN</u>

Biotin is one of the many B-Vitamins that have been receiving renewed interest for its prophylactic value in combating hair loss. When biotin is utilized in hair care products the elasticity of the hair's cortex is greatly enhanced, thereby preventing breakage. Furthermore the actual hair cuticle is thickened providing a fuller appearance because of the increased diameter of each hair shaft. This dual therapeutic action upon the follicle gives it added protection from free radicals and increases the hair's natural sheen.

To isolate more upon the vitamin itself it is a noted growth stimulant and necessary for fatty acid synthesis in the body. In replicated studies of biotin combined with niacin (vitamin B-3), hair growth was established. The ingredients were applied in gel form. In one of the more well-known studies in which biotin was utilized ninety percent of the participants involved showed a marked reduction in hair loss to fully normal levels. This was accomplished by using biotin only twice a week. The subjects in this case included both sexes and ranged in age from twenty to seventy. Hair regrowth also occurred in seventy-five percent of the tested subjects. As this study and many others have established, you simply can't go wrong with biotin!

- **We definitely recommend any shampoo or conditioner**

containing biotin. **When purchasing these ingredients it is preferable to look for biotin and niacin in the same product to increase their potency. Noted specialist, Dr. Edward Settel has done extensive research regarding the value of biotin in the treatment of baldness.**

- **To increase the effectiveness of biotin products one should leave the shampoos or conditioners on the scalp for at least three minutes before rinsing. When using biotin conditioners you should towel the scalp before applying.**

- **Results from utilizing biotin products should become evident in two to four weeks. Hair loss should decrease substantially.**

PRODUCTS CONTAINING BIOTIN

1. **Biotene H-24 Hair Care Products**
   http://www.gnc.com
2. **Nexus Biotin Shampoo and Biotin Cream**
3. **Nature's Plus Ultra Hair Sustained Release**
   http://www.evitamins.com
   http://www.vitacost.com
   http://www.swansonvitamins.com
4. **Nioxin Shampoos**
5. **Nisim Hair Loss Shampoo**
   http://www.nisim.com
   http://www.skin-beauty.com
6. **GNC (General Nutrition Stores) Biotin Products**
7. **Mill Creek Biotin Products**
   http://www.drvita.com
   http://www.ihealthtree.com
8. **Joico Clinicure System**
   http://www.ariva.com
   http://www.brightonbeautysupply.com
9. **Jason Naturals Biotin Shampoo and Conditioner**
   http://www.vitacost.com
10. **Nature's Gate Biotin Treatment Shampoo**
    http://www.drvita.com
11. **Puritan's Pride**
    http://www.puritan.com

12.   Bio-Genesis Bioteine H-3 Gel
http://www.headstartvitamins.com

BLACK SEED OIL

Of all documented cases of herbal usage black seed oil probably can claim the longest history. Scientifically known as Nigella Sativa its usage dates back to the Assyrian Empire. Its popularity was further enhanced when the prophet Muhammad proclaimed "black seed has healing for all illnesses except death." Still today in the Middle East it is known as the "seed of blessing."

To amplify on what makes this plant so popular we must first look at the various compounds it contains. The oil itself is a rich source of vitamins, minerals, essential fatty acids, eight amino acids, carotenoids, monosaccharides, polysaccharides, sterols, plus 100 other substances some unique only to black seed. Even though considerable U.S. research has been conducted on black seed in the past ten years it still perplexes many researchers. The mystery lies in whether the plant accomplishes its healing mechanisms through the various herbal combinations working in unison or whether particular ingredients are triggering them.

Scientists refer to black seed oil as an immunomodulator because it has the ability to enhance an under active immune system or "quiet" and overactive one. Many recent studies have shown black seed capable of increasing T-Helper cells, stimulating bone marrow cells, escalating interferon production, energizing antibody producing B-cells, and even attacking tumors directly. Add to that the fact it is used to treat psoriasis, arthritis, diabetes, and allergies and you have a very potent drug.

In relation to hair loss the oil has been used for years in the Middle East as a hair loss antagonist and stimulant for growing hair. Since the oil is rich in polysaccharides, essential fatty acids, vasodilators, and naturally occurring DHT inhibitors, as we've mentioned, it certainly wouldn't hurt hair growth. The most interesting fact about black seed oil is that some leading hair experts claim hair loss is directly related to over-activity of the immune system. Since black seed is a quoted immune modulator it may externally reverse some of the cell activity directly related to hair loss.

SOURCES FOR BLACK SEED OIL

1. **Sweet Sunnah Black Seed Oil and Henna Shampoo**
    http://www.sweetsunnah.com
    http://www.black-seed-oil.com

BLACK TEA EXTRACTS

The old saying "you are what you eat" is more likely "you are what you drink" when it pertains to androgenetic alopecia. Amazingly the ingredient black tea is slightly more potent than Propecia in reducing the bad DHT that is rated as one of the causative factors in pattern hair loss. In fact with scientific studies conducted at Harvard University the actual reduction percentages for DHT are Propecia by 71% and black tea by an amount of 72%. Plus natural black tea escalates the amount of testosterone in our bodies which commonly declines with the presence of pattern baldness. Propecia on the other hand does not do that. Furthermore black tea enhances the strength of your blood vessel walls which reduces the chance of strokes and cardiovascular events. This alone is enough to make you rethink what type of beverages you should be ingesting. Really the only negative factor is using caffeine in abundance. This can be countered by using decaffeinated blends that are only slightly less potent.

As for side effects there are relatively none. With Propecia on the other hand side effects such as decreased libido, gynecomastia (breast enlargement), and psycho/neurological disturbances have been reported. Quite the contrary with black tea none of this occurs and it does increase the sex drive in many. Whether this is related to the caffeine or other components of black tea has never been fully tested.

Other tests have shown that the likely explanation for the increase in androgenetic alopecia among rural Oriental males and females exposed to Western living is probably related to the reduction of soy and black tea in their diets.

SOURCES FOR BLACK TEA EXTRACTS

1. **Tetley Iced and Regular Tea Bags**
2. **Lipton Iced and Regular Tea Bags**
3. **Solaray Black Tea Extract**
    http://www.totaldiscountvitamins.com

http://www.vitacost.com
http://www.vitaglo.com

BLUEBERRIES

What's the top power food for preventing hair loss? Well most would have never guessed it is the lowly blueberry. Long recognized as one of the leading anti-oxidants this berry packs quite a punch. Why is it so beneficial for hair loss sufferers? Well the answer lays in the old saying "if it's good for the eyes it's definitely good for hair loss." The simple reason behind that is this berry contains sizable amounts of Lutein and zeaxanthin which are excellent for your vision. The bottom line being is this fruit promotes blood circulation in even the minutest capillaries which is essential for hair growth. Add to that the fact it reduces LDL which is the bad type of cholesterol and you have quite a berry.

To tell you a little bit more about the blueberry it is a perennial indigenous to North America and was used by the Indians long before Europeans arrived on the coastline. In fact it was a daily staple among many tribes for hundreds of years. The Indians quickly learned it could be dried and ground and eaten at a later date without losing its potency. It was also used as a preservative.

Extracts of the blueberry contain resveratrol, pterostilbene, flavanols, tannins, proanthocyanidins, and anthocyanins. The two latter ingredients being linked to cures for cancer. Pterostilbene on the other hand is similar to resveratrol but may have future value in reversing the cognitive decline often seen in Alzheimer's disease.

SOURCES FOR BLUEBERRIES

1. **Blueberry Juice**
2. **Blueberry Supplements**

BROCCOLI

One vegetable long touted by juicers as cure for pattern hair loss is now receiving renewed exposure as doing just that. Much of the research has centered on unique chemicals in broccoli that have the ability to ward off and even destroy cancers. One chemical in particular known as sulforaphane has shown an ability to halt the deadly bacterium helicobacter pylori which is chiefly responsible for stomach ulcers and other deadly forms of stomach cancers. To further exemplify its uniqueness sulfforphane when isolated was able to totally eradicate antibiotic resistant helicobacter pylori.

In relation to male and female pattern hair loss chemicals in broccoli are potent DHT inhibitors. The true fact though is when broccoli is digested it combines with enzymes that accelerate the function of the liver. With this acceleration of liver function, which decreases with the aging process, free radicals and bad DHT are now properly eliminated from the body. Interestingly enough Chinese medicine largely associates pattern baldness with impaired functioning of the liver. On the other hand those that specialize in hair research readily point out every vitamin and mineral component necessary for hair and bone growth can be found in broccoli.

Broccoli is a member of the cabbage family, and is closely related to cauliflower.

SOURCES FOR BROCCOLI

1.   **Many people find raw broccoli and cauliflower are excellent snacks that curb the appetite. Low in calories and delicious with your favorite dips it's truly a wondrous food.**

BURDOCK ROOT

Burdock Root or Arctium Lappa is a carrot like biennial herb grown in China, Europe, and the United States. It is employed as a popular folk medicine around the world and is consumed as a vegetable in Japan where it is called "gobo".

The extracts of the seeds have has been used for years as a popular cure to purify blood, halt hair loss, treat gout and arthritis, and cure skin diseases such as acne and psoriasis. In India and Russia it is utilized to treat various forms of cancer. The Chinese though have long believed it to be an effective aphrodisiac, useful in treating impotence and sterility.

The volatile oils of burdock seed are said to be an effective diaphoretic, used in inducing sweating as an aid in neutralizing and eliminating toxins from the body. This activity is widely utilized by herbal practitioners in the treatment of liver problems, gallstones, flu, and to support the kidneys in filtering acids from the blood stream.

Studies show burdock has a high content of minerals especially iron. Data also indicates the root is a source of carbohydrates in particular inulin. The oils though tend to be the most sought after agent in the herb.

Burdock oil when applied to the scalp exhibits anti-bacterial and antifungal properties. It does appear the oils have some DHT inhibiting qualities along with the vasodilator effects it can induce within the hair follicles.

If you desire to use burdock it can be purchased in the oil-based form and applied to the thinning areas of the scalp after shampooing. Once you do this let the hair dry normally until you desire to apply again. Many people claimed it has helped their hair loss problems greatly but it has never found overwhelming acceptance.

- **Burdock Oil can be directly added to shampoos to achieve its benefits.**

SOURCES FOR BURDOCK ROOT

1. **Mostly found in vitamin, herb, and nutritional stores.**
2. **Herbavita Nettle And Burdock Shampoo**
   http://www.vitaminlife.com
3. **Aveda Scalp Benefits Balancing Shampoo**
   http://www.aveda.com
4. **Nature's Gate Rainwater Herbal Shampoo**
   http://www.vitamin-provider.com
5. **Floraleads Burdock Root Hair Oil**
   http://floraleads.com
6. **Max Green Alchemy Hair Rescue Shampoo**
   http://www.maxgreenalchemy.com

NATURAL HAIR LOSS INGREDIENTS GROUP C

CAFFEINE

Strange as it may seem Eastern European researchers have made claims that coffee grounds may be beneficial in combating hair loss. Even though it has long been established that the components of all teas, especially green tea, are beneficial in retarding hair loss coffee itself has never been researched as a retardant to pattern baldness. According to German scientists the ingredient that makes this possible is the actual caffeine. The caveat here is the caffeine must be applied externally. Consumption of this beverage, that so many people find delicious, will not do the trick.

- **Caffeine shampoo can be made relatively easily by adding just a couple of tablespoons of ground coffee to an unscented shampoo and shaking. This combination should only be used once a week followed with a good conditioner.**

- **European researchers claim caffeine is most beneficial when left on the scalp at least two minutes. This allows the active ingredient to fully penetrate the follicle and work its magic.**

SOURCES FOR CAFFEINE

1. **Found in any grocery store.**
2. **Thicker Fuller Hair Revitalizing Shampoo with Caffeine – Widespread availability in retail stores such as CVS.**
3. **Garnier Fructis Fall Fight Fortifying Shampoo**
4. **Goldwell for Men Dualsenses Thickening Shampoo**
   http://www.beautyencounter.com
   http://www.bestbeautyboutique.com
5. **Dove Men Care Fortifying Shampoo Aqua Impact**
6. **Keune Care Line Derma Activating Shampoo and Lotion**
   http://www.beautycarechoices.com
   http://www.sleekhair.com
7. **Capillus Shampoos and Treatments**
   http://www.cannabis-cosmetics.com
8. **ThermaScalp Natural Scalp Therapy**
   http://www.greensations.com
9. **DS Laboratories Revita**
   http://www.gnc.com
10. **Alpecin Shampoo**

http://www.alpecin.com
http://www.pampered.com
http://www.boots.com

11.   **Plantur 39**
http://www.plantur39.com
http://www.expresschemist.co.uk

12.   **Davines Natural Tech Energizing Shampoo**
http://us.davines.com
http://www.blushbeautystore.com

13.   **Logona Shampoo Age Energy Organic Caffeine & Goji Berry**
http://www.luckyvitamin.com

CAPSAICIN-CAYENNE PEPPER

This hot biting herb is regaining popularity after a brief fling in the 80's. Researchers are beginning to take note that the active ingredient (capsicum) of this herb is an extremely powerful stimulant when applied topically or taken internally. The herb being a rich source of vitamin A, niacin (a growth factor), and vitamin C can stimulate blood flow in the particular area applied. Interestingly enough one of the most talked about baldness cures outside the United States contains the active ingredient capsaicin. Claims have been made this formula called Fabao 101D has results that far exceed those of minoxidil. Even though the company's research is weak by American standards it has extremely high sales figures. Leading international corporations are quickly taking notice of this and you can expect to see compounds possibly entering the market shortly, as hair regrowth solutions. Interest also stems from the fact that there is no known systemic absorption when applied topically, so side effects are few if any.

Our position though is for individuals to look for OTC hair care products containing cayenne pepper in nutritional stores. Since the herb can certainly cause histamine release it's unquestionably a tool for combating hair loss. Always remember though if you decide to take cayenne pepper in pill form it can agitate an ulcer.

- **One method of usage for capsaicin is to apply the lotion formulas sparingly to the forehead to create a vasodilator effect. Then follow with other hair loss treatments. Cayenne Pepper may also be mixed with the shampoos you may already be using.**

- Always observe caution when using any form of pepper near your eyes.

- Powdered or finely ground Cayenne Pepper can be integrated any shampoo of your choice. Just remember to shake thoroughly to dissolve the ingredients.

- Capsaicin has been linked to relieving the symptoms of arthritis, preventing blood clots, lowering blood sugar, and reducing cluster headaches. But quite the opposite of what you might expect most people use this herb for weight loss. Apparently the derivative capsaicin somehow resets the fat thermostat in our bodies enabling it to burn more brown fat.

PRODUCTS CONTAINING CAPSAICIN

1. Various products found at local nutritional stores.
2. Chile's Romero & Espinocilla Shampoo
   http://www.justbeautysupplies.com
3. Hair Vite Chili Pepper Shampoo
   http://www.nutriwell.net
4. ReviveTH Shampoo
   http://www.haircareusa.com
   http://www.hairproductsgalore.com
5. Spanish Garden Pepper Treatment Shampoo
   http://pennherb.com
   http://gardenpharmacynj.com
6. Sante Natural Invigorating Chili Pepper Shampoo
7. Grow Conditioner
   http://www.growshampoo.com
8. ThermaScalp Natural Scalp Therapy
   http://www.greensations.com
9. Peppar Shampoo and Conditioner
   http://www.cachebeauty.com/palmbeach.htm
10. Cayenne Pepper - Local Supermarket spice sections.
11. Nature's Way Hair and Skin Formula
    http://www.drvita.com
    http://www.vitacost.com
12. Alter EGO Energizing Shampoo
    http://www.beautyofnewyork.com

CASTOR OIL

Castor Oil is an interesting ingredient that you will find in better hair care products. The oil itself has many of the qualities of sebum but does not lend itself to clogging scalp pores. The active agent in castor oil is ricnoleic acid. Applied to the scalp it reduces inflammation and lubricates the skin and hair. For years the oil has been used to retard hair loss but no substantial evidence has ever validated the claim. Even though ricnoleic acid has known anti-oxidant properties that would be beneficial to the scalp the research is spotty regarding this acid. Never less it should not be ignored as hair loss preventative in finer hair care products.

SOURCES FOR CASTOR OIL

1. **Scruples Hair Care Products**
2. **Olde Jamaica Vitamin Black Castor Oil Shampoo and Conditioner**
   http://www.oldejamaica.com
3. **Cranberry Lane Natural Hair Care Products**
   http://www.cranberrylane.com/
4. **Castor Oil**
   http://www.baar.com
   http://www.nutriwell.net
5. **Roffler Hair Care Products**
6. **Castor Oil Shampoo**
   http://www.etsy.com
   http://www.houseofbeautyworld.com
7. **Schwarzkopf Professional Bonacure For Men Phytobiogin Tonic, Shampoo, and Conditioner**
   http://www.sleekhair.com
8. **Kuz Hair Loss Control Cream**
   http://bluebeez.com
   http://www.beautyofnewyork.com
9. **Rene Furterer Forticea Stimulating Shampoo**
   http://www.lovelyskin.com
   http://www.evabeauty.com

CHROMIUM

Chromium is probably one of the few minerals that none of us get enough of in our diet. The mineral itself helps us turn carbohydrates into glucose, an important energy source. Chromium may also help in relieving the symptoms of hypoglycemia, prevent some people from developing diabetes, and protect the heart and arteries. Sugar intake along with stress increases the secretion of chromium from the body. Even though the suggested government intake is between 50 and 200 mcg a day, few individuals ingest over 25 mcg a day. Herbalists report that by taking between 200 and 600 mcg of this mineral daily you can prevent baldness.

- **We personally do not recommend exceeding the typical 200 mcg dosage.**

SOURCES FOR CHROMIUM

1. **An excellent source for this nutrient is Chromium Picolate. It can be found in the vitamin sections of most stores. There are many versions of this nutrient but you need not pay a high price for it to be effective. The nutrient itself can be found in many good multi-vitamins such as Centrum at Walmart or Walgreens.**

CIMETIDINE-TAGAMET

Cimetidine is known as histamine blocker. These drugs were developed to control symptoms associated with ulcers and excess acids in the digestive track. The trade name of this particular drug being Tagamet. It is also popularly known as an acid reducer.

Tagamet has been associated with DHT lowering and anti-androgen capabilities that can prevent hair loss. Research though is limited in this matter. Since Tagamet is sold specifically for acid reduction limited use for any other purpose would be advisable. It is sold OTC (over the counter). Undocumented reports indicate that use of Tagamet once or twice weekly in the 200 mcg. formulation may be completely satisfactory for stemming hair loss.

- **Tagamet is sold about everywhere now. Stronger versions of the drug (400mg.) are available by prescription. Cimetidine is usually cheaper when purchased this way but over the counter products can serve the same purpose. Furthermore not all acid blockers possess anti-androgenic capabilities, if you're**

34

wondering. Pill splitters can be utilized with the OTC versions of Tagamet to quarter the tabs.

SOURCES FOR CIMETIDINE-TAGAMET

1. **Walmart Stores**
2. **Most Drug Stores**

COLD WATER TREATMENT

A recent Canadian study was able to counteract hair loss simply using cold water rinses on the scalp after shampooing. Supposedly the drop in temperature generated by the icy water is able to inhibit the thinning process, when used over a two to four week period of time. Interestingly the theories were derived from chemotherapy treatments designed to counteract the effects of cancer. Since this is probably one of the cheapest remedies to experiment with it couldn't hurt to try it out. Anecdotal evidence is abundant but since the original study lacked a significant number of participants the validity of the results is open to debate.

COLD WATER SOURCES

1. **Ordinary cold tap water.**

COLON CLEANSING

Proponents of colon cleansing claim since there is no one single cause for hair loss, but a chain of events, the only way to treat thinning hair is by normalizing the body's various systems. In other words thinning hair is not just a problem of the scalp, it is a problem of the whole body and how it functions. To best do this you must first cleanse the body of excess wastes, poisons, parasites, and toxins that have accumulated through the years. Once you've engaged in these cleansings often enough you can then return to exercising regularly, eating a healthy diet with more fruits and vegetables, and reducing your fat and meat consumption. To sum it up by putting your system on a normal footing you're likely to reduce your thinning hair and grow new hair whether or not its cause is medical or genetic. Gurus of these methods recommend simple bowel cleansing for eradicating your hair loss problems but they do offer an array of cleansing techniques. This assortment can include the removal of mercury based fillings in your mouth all the way up to gallbladder, parasite, and liver cleanses. For the typical individual simple colon cleanses will suffice when you're dealing with hair loss. At worst you'll likely experience greater energy, lose weight, and see noticeable improvements in your skin and hair.

Bottom line colon cleansing is one of many alternative treatments that treat the body as a whole to alleviate various disorders such as hair loss. As even the most elite doctors have learned the most targeted of therapies can fail because the body must be treated in its entirety to eliminate the problem. This is particularly true with diseases such as cancer that can rapidly metastasize because treatment was confined to a particular area.

- **Numerous colon cleansing products are available in the marketplace today. Large retailers carry the largest variety and entertain the best prices.**

SOURCES FOR COLON CLEANSING

1. **Walgreens**
2. **Walmart**

CRUDE OIL

This may seem like a strange one but for years North American Indians have use variations of crude oil to combat diseases of the scalp and hair loss. The reality is that crude oil makes an excellent cleanser for the scalp and has excellent antiseptic qualities. Canadian studies have shown when properly formulated crude oil can induce and control hair loss. It has been suggested crude oil un-blocks plugged hair follicles to induce the hair growth. The most likely scenario though is that it either initiates changes in the upper area of the hair follicle or creates a histamine release that induces the growth. Either way it does seem promising. Just make sure that it isn't to irritating to your scalp. If it is use a hair conditioner to combat the dryness.

SOURCES FOR CRUDE OIL HAIR CARE PRODUCTS

1. **Herald Tar Shampoo**
2. **Denorex Shampoo**
3. **Neutrogena T/Gel Shampoo**
4. **Baar Pennsylvania Crude Oil Shampoo**

http://www.baar.com
5. **Heritage Crudoleum Shampoos and Conditioners –
Limited availability heavy demand.**
http://www.caycecures.com
http://www.vitaminbuddy.com
http://www.taoofherbs.com

NATURAL HAIR LOSS INGREDIENTS GROUP D

DUTASTERIDE

Dutasteride is a medication marketed by Smith, Glaxo, and Kline as a treatment for benign prostatic hyperplasia. Dutasteride belongs to a class of drugs called 5-alpha-reductase inhibitors. These types of drugs block the conversion of enzymes that transform testosterone into dihydrotestosterone (DHT). It is basically a cousin of Propecia (Finasteride) the well-known hair growth pill from the same manufacturer. Marketed in the United States as Avodart it is also sold under the names Avidart, Avolve, Duagen, Dutas, Dutagen, and Duprost in the worldwide community. Dutasteride has been reported as being significantly more effective than Propecia for growing hair. The comparative doses between the two are .5 (mg) for Avodart and 1 (mg) for Propecia.

The reason why we report on Dutasteride is because of its wide availability in the "gray market" similar to Propecia and Proscar. The main side effects of Avodart are erectile dysfunction, gynecomastia, decreased libido, and ejaculation disorders, which are similar to the problems reported with Propecia. Also the half-life of Propecia is considerably shorter than with Avodart therefore the duration of side effects would be longer. Dutasteride was tested at a 2.5(mg) dosage, which is five times the dosage they currently sell. Reported side effects for this level were 3-4% where with Propecia it was 1-2%.

- **The plus side of Dutasteride is the long half-life. Instead of using a daily dosage, similar to Propecia, many people report using it only once weekly for hair growth or to maintain the hair they already have. The half-life of Avodart, or how long it stays in the bloodstream, is 240 hours or 10 days. On the other hand at most the half-life of Propecia is 4 days.**

- **Smith, Glaxo, and Kline did discontinue testing of Dutasteride in phase two of their testing without a reported reason. There are normally three phases of testing. Speculation is that since they already had one successful hair loss drug in the marketplace they did not want to introduce a competing product. Since that point in 2006 they have reinstated the phase three testing.**

- **Dutasteride can be purchased within the "gray market" for about as much as generic Proscar. If you're using dutasteride based upon a weekly or biweekly schedule the price is considerably cheaper than Proscar and Propecia.**

- **This drug is not prescribed for women.**

SOURCES FOR DUTASTERIDE

1. **Your Local Pharmacy**
2. **https://www.northdrugmart.com**
3. **http://www.planetdrugsdirect.com**
4. **http://www.canadadrugs.com**

NATURAL HAIR LOSS INGREDIENTS GROUP E

EGG BASED SOLUTIONS

Many people claim the solution for hair loss may sit right in your local grocery store. Long used as a conditioning base in finer hair care products, eggs contain numerous vitamins and minerals. Add to that substantial amounts of protein and you have the building blocks for an excellent scalp treatment. Plus eggs are the standard by which all other protein sources are measured. The reason for this is that eggs contain all of the essential amino acids in proper proportion for human nutrition. So it's not unusual for hair conditioning products to derive their ingredients from this dairy product.

If you want to try out this solution, to retard hair loss, we have included a sample recipe below. Remember there are dozens of ways people make egg based shampoos and conditioners and they abound on the Internet. So don't think you're married to just this one.

Recipe for Egg Shampoo

1 egg
1 tsp. olive oil
1 tsp. lemon juice
1 T. castile soap or mild unscented shampoo
1/2 C. water

Combine all ingredients in a blender and whip until smooth. Use shampoo immediately, and follow up with a hair rinse. Save any remaining shampoo in the refrigerator and use the next day.

SOURCES FOR EGG BASED SOLUTIONS

1. **Mario Badescu Skin Care**
   http://www.mariobadescu.com
2. **Organix Nourishing Coconut Milk Shampoo**
3. **Keune Egg Shampoo**
   http://www.beautysupplysource.com
   http://www.beautysupplycanada.com
4. **Phytologie Phytorhum Fortifying Shampoo**
   http://www.belairbeauty.com
   http://www.fragrancesaver.com

EMU OIL

One ingredient that is receiving more and more publicity as an actual hair-restorer is Emu oil. This extract is derived from the flightless Emu bird indigenous to the Australian Outback. For years Aborigines of these regions used the oil as a moisturizer, antiseptic, analgesic rub, burn treatment, and for muscular pains. Many professional sports teams now make use of this oil for a myriad of aches and sprains.

This oil's rare property is that it is one of the few substances with the molecular weight to penetrate deep into the skin. Doing so allows it to stimulate the blood flow to areas where applied. The advantage of this is that the healing process is noticeably quickened and collagen production is considerably enhanced. The added plus is that this ingredient is completely non-toxic and doesn't possess the usual greasiness of most oils. Also by virtue of its absorbability into the dermis, other ingredients are able to hitch a ride on it for added benefits. Aloe Vera in particular.

In regard to hair loss, tests conducted on rodents in 1995 with this oil indicated very positive results in regard to hair regrowth. Astoundingly the hair growth was thicker than what was previously observed before using the oil. Many exotic hair restoration formulas use this oil as their chief ingredient.

If you would like to make use of this oil it should be applied to thinning areas of the scalp before retiring and washed out in the morning. Application is required only once a day. Results if obtained should be expected within two to eight weeks.

- **Emu oil is particularly high in some of the essential fatty acids. Notably linolenic acid and oleic acid which are known anti-inflammatory agents.**

- **Reports are that Emu oil has the capability to darken graying hair. If you are going to see results it takes about two months of usage.**

- **Two newer studies by very reputable researchers claim that Emu oil may be one of the most effective ingredients for growing hair found to date.**

SOURCES FOR EMU OIL

1. **Long View Farms**
   http://www.longviewfarms.com/
2. **NuGen Emu Oil Shampoo**
   http://www.salonweb.com
3. **Emusing Secrets**
   http://www.emusingsecrets.com
4. **Maple Springs**
   www.maplesprings.com
5. **Accelerate Shampoo (Black Hair Care)**
   http://www.salonweb.com
   http://www.exoticallure.com
6. **General Nutrition Stores**
7. **Emu Oil Minnesota**
   http://emuoilminnesota.com

8. **Blue Spring Hair Healthy Shampoo with Emu Oil**
   http://www.bluespringwellness.com
9. **Uniquely Emu Products**
   http://www.uniquelyemu.com/
10. **Healthy Hair Plus**
    http://www.healthyhairplus.com
11. **Arizona Emu Oil Shampoo Bar**
    http://www.arizonaemuoil.com
12. **Omega Emu Products**
    http://www.worldofhair.com/hair/omega.htm

ESSENTIAL FATTY ACIDS

One group of nutrients often overlooked and greatly underestimated, for halting hair loss and promoting regrowth on the scalp, are the essential fatty acids. These fatty acids encompass a broad spectrum which includes omega (inolenic acid), omega 3 (linoleic acid), black current, borage, evening primrose, and fish oil. The importance of these oils derives from the fact they are necessary for the production of prostaglandins in our bodies. Prostaglandins are hormone like substances that regulate most of our physiological processes. These functions include the cardiovascular, immune, pulmonary, reproductive, and digestive systems.

Researchers claim that these fatty acids are able to curb the production of biochemicals which form in the body when it is placed under emotional and physical duress. Interestingly enough practitioners of natural medicine (homeopaths) claim these stress bi-products have a greater effect on hair growth than one might realize. Parenthetically studies done of Rogaine at Tulane University cited that even minute amounts of stress might be more of a causative factor in hair loss than once was theorized. This being the case, practitioners of natural medicine often prescribe a treatment of these fatty acids and other herbs that lessen the corresponding tolls brought on the body by this strain. And if you're wondering many anti-anxiety drugs do reduce hair loss, but we are certainly not recommending that course of action for the apparent reasons.

The body furthermore cannot produce essential fatty acids so they must either come from our diet or supplements. Research indicates that only about twenty five percent of people in Western cultures ever obtain the daily requirements of these fatty acids. This being the consequence of most of us consuming a greater amount of processed food than wild foods.

Probably one of the more effective fatty acids is evening primrose oil, which contains gamma linolenic acid (GLA). Hundreds of studies have indicated gamma linolenic acid is helpful in relieving a wide range of ailments related to the hair, skin, and nails. This assortment of ills does include hair loss, acne, dermatitis, eczema, arthritis, obesity, and fungus infections.

Flaxseed Oil is probably one of the better sources for the Omega 3's. Omega 3's tending to be one of the fatty acids most lacking in the diets of western cultures.

Borage on the other hand is a vegetable oil derived from the seeds of a blue flowering plant found exclusively in Europe. Physicians in these areas often prescribe the oil's extract to counteract inflammation and restore adrenal gland functions. As a whole the seed oil of this plant has the largest concentration of GLA's but it tends to be more expensive than evening primrose oil.

Flaxseed oil, black current, and fish oils also contain greater variations of the previously listed fatty acids.

Fascinatingly enough some companies are selling products that combine fish oils and combinations of these GLA's and Omega's to prevent hair loss and regrow hair. You can experiment with many of these fine herbs on your own. By doing so you can save yourself a considerable amount of money and see what's appropriate for you at the same time.

- **Many people probably aren't aware that the extracts of the herb saw palmetto contain about eighty-five to ninety percent pure fatty acids. This is partially why the constituents of this plant are reportedly effective against baldness. And remember these fatty acids are naturally derived as opposed to pharmaceutical products.**

- **Many Scandinavian products that utilize fish oils claim great success in combating hair loss and establishing regrowth. Interestingly enough many of these exact same nutrients can be purchased in vitamin and nutrition** stores. **Considering the fact that quite a few of these companies are charging up to two hundred dollars for a month's supply your own savings could be considerable. Fish oils can contain a variety of fatty acids beneficial for many medical conditions.**

- **Salmon, fish, and flaxseed oils tend to be the more popular products for obtaining essential fatty acids to prevent hair loss.**

SOURCES FOR ESSENTIAL FATTY ACIDS

1. **GNC Stores - These stores have an excellent variety of fatty acids in supplement form.**
2. **Walmart Stores - Excellent prices for Borage and Evening Primrose.**
3. **Walgreens**
4. **CVS Drug Stores**
5. **Jason Hemp Shampoo and Conditioner**
6. **Hair Fitness Nutrient Shampoo and Conditioner**
   http://www.healthandbodyfitness.com
7. **Aubrey Organics Rosa Mosqueta Rose Hip Herbal Conditioner**
   http://www.aubrey-organics.com
8. **Aubrey Organics Sea Buckthorn Leave In Conditioner**
   http://www.vitaminlife.com
   http://www.bewellstaywell.com
9. **Mastey Traite Moisturizing Shampoo**
10. **Onesta Shampoo and Conditioner**
    http://www.hairproducts4me.com
11. **Essential Fatty Acids**
    http://www.drvita.com

NATURAL HAIR LOSS INGREDIENTS GROUP F

FENUGREEK

Fenugreek has been a prized healing agent since medieval times. Once prescribed for respiratory complaints and waning sexual desires, it is no longer considered the cure-all it once was.

The secret of this alkaloid plant lies in the seeds, which contain mucilage. Mucilage is a slimy, oily substance that soothes and protects sore or inflamed tissues, especially those of the skin.

This unusual agent seems to have a synergetic effect on hair follicles when combined with the B-Vitamins. Though it remains a mystery as to why this occurs, European research indicates the combination can be a legitimate hair restorer. Apparently this combination of vitamins and herbs create a potent DHT inhibitor that encourages hair growth. The alkaloids could also be a source of nitric oxides, which may be a causative factor for the growth. American research has not established this. Various U.S. patents utilizing these alkaloids, as hair growth stimulants, are on file though.

- **Dr. Peter Proctor a leading authority on hair loss maintains that the use of nitric oxides can stimulate hair growth.**

SOURCES FOR FENUGREEK

1. **Fenugreek is not your typical supplement so you will usually only find it at Vitamin and Nutrition stores.**
2. **B vitamins can be found about everywhere.**
3. **Arcon Tisane**
4. **Origenere Shampoo for Thinning Hair**
   http://www.origenere.com
5. **Folligro Hair Loss Shampoo**
   http://www.buybeauty.com
   http://drkowalski.stores.yahoo.net
   http://buybeauty.com
6. **Folli-Cleanse Shampoo**
   http://healthyhairplus.com/
   http://www.hairenergizer.com
7. **Better Botanicals Neem Care Shampoo**
   http://www.betterbotanicals.com
8. **Himalaya Herbals Protein Shampoo**
   http://www.herbal-provider.com
   http://www.haircareherbal.com
9. **IHT 9 Herbal Hair Regrowth Shampoo**
   http://www.iht9.com

FOLLIGEN

Folligen is a mail order product sold by Skin Biology. Skin Biology is an international corporation marketing various wounds healing products to the medical fields. The creator of this product is one of the original inventors of Iamin Gel. Folligen itself employs a copper peptone and saw palmetto as part of its base. The product does have anti-androgen effects upon the scalp. The reason we recognize this product is that it is available now and is considered safe. Reports are that this product is as effective as minoxidil. At a cost of about seventeen dollars a tube or twenty five dollars for the spray solution the contents should last you two to three months. Individual accounts also indicate that this product may be much better for the frontal hairline than minoxidil.

The makers of Folligen follow a different strategy as to the causes of pattern baldness. Rather than being the result of the by-products of testosterone, their belief is that dermal damage may be the antagonist. Skin Biology points to the fact that many people with high testosterone levels never experience hair loss, as evidence of their theories. Clinical tests of Folligen's active ingredients show that they are able to improve the scalp's mantle, thereby improving the quality of hair follicle reproduction. It is a patented product.

The suggested use pattern for this product is four times a week. It does come in a cream formula for the hairline and lotion for denser areas of the scalp.

- **To use Folligen a thin film of the cream or lotion should be applied to the scalp four times a week, before retiring at night. Some users also apply minoxidil at the same time. This can be done by first applying the minoxidil and allowing it to dry. Then administer the Folligen. Folligen should be rinsed from the hair upon rising.**

- **Folligen's price does drop when ordered in quantity from Skin Biology. It is also offered in a competitively priced package with minoxidil. Prices and products are subject to change based upon demand.**

ORDERING INFORMATION FOR FOLLIGEN

1. **Folligen**
   http://hairloss101.com
   http://onlyhairloss.com
2. **Skin Biology**
   http://store.reverseskinaging.com
3. **Therapro Folligen for Women**
   http://www.theraprohair.com
   http://www.evabeauty.com

NATURAL HAIR LOSS INGREDIENTS GROUP G

GARLIC

The botanical name for this herb is Allium sativum, and it belongs to the Allium genus of the Alliaceae family. It is well known for its anti-fungal antibacterial, antiviral, and anti-parasitic properties. The chemical composition of this herb includes minerals, enzymes, flavonoids, plus the A and B vitamins. Some of the included minerals are calcium, copper, iron, manganese, phosphorus, potassium and selenium. Overall it is a good source of protein and adds tremendously to the culinary experience as either a seasoning or condiment. As for medicinal purposes garlic supplementation has been shown to reduce cholesterol and has benefit in lowering blood pressure. Garlic is known for causing halitosis.

What garlic is best known for is the sulfur type substances found within it. Remarkably this herb contains over 80 of these compounds which are highly beneficial to the scalp.

As a hair loss aid it has been shown to have benefit in the treatment of alopecia areata in particular. Considerable anecdotal evidence does indicate garlic shampoos and supplements do seem to lessen hair loss and stimulate some hair growth when used over an extended period of time.

- **If you are going to use garlic hair care products or supplements it is advisable to use unscented or deodorized brands.**

SOURCES FOR GARLIC

1. **Nutrine Garlic Shampoo**
   http://www.justbeautysupplies.com
   http://www.beautyofnewyork.com
   http://www.vermontcountrystore.com
2. **Eko Garlic Shampoo**
3. **Nora Ross Garlic Shampoo**
   http://www.noraross.com
4. **E Voss Keratin Plus Garlic Shampoo**
   http://www.evossdna.com
5. **Alter Ego Garlic Shampoo**
   http://www.bluebeez.com

GRAPE SEED EXTRACT

One nutrient we absolutely don't want to ignore, because of its increased availability, is grape seed extract. Reported to have fifty times the anti-oxidant capabilities of vitamins E and C, it is unquestionably one of the more potent free radical scavengers available today. The extract itself allows the body's cells to cope with numerous chemical threats that would otherwise impair its health and vitality. It does this by utilizing various procyanidolic oligomers often referred to as procyanidins.

Ironically the grape seed extract industry had its birth more or less in explaining the so-called French paradox. This contradiction was encountered in France when it was observed that many wine drinkers had exceedingly high cholesterol levels but low incidences of cardiovascular disease. Scientists had long known that alcohol usage did increase cholesterol levels, which could lead to heart disease, but they were baffled as to why many Frenchmen showed just the opposite. Ultimately the answer was traced to the procyandins in the skins and seeds of grapes. Voila, grape seed extract.

Interestingly enough even though no formal studies have been done establishing grape seed extract as a hair loss antagonist, discoveries in other areas have been promising. Grape seed extract has been shown to halt hair loss when the body has been exposed to harsh chemotherapy and acetaminophen damage. Along with enhancing the functions of the liver and capillaries, testing shows it may even kill a variety of cancer cells. It does this while increasing the vitality of the body's cells, at the same time.

Our feeling is that you simply shouldn't be ignoring this extract as a part of any arsenal to prevent hair loss. At worse this nutrient could lend itself to improving your cardiovascular system, the liver's functioning, and potentially fights off some cancers. Plus it's shown itself to be safe and devoid of most side effects.

SOURCES FOR GRAPE SEED EXTRACT

1. **Schifft's Grape Seed Extract - Walmart Stores**
2. **Sundown Herbals Grape Seed Extract Complex - Walmart Stores**
3. **GNC Stores**
4. **CVS Drugstores**
5. **Phytocyane Revitalizing Shampoo for Women**
    http://www.beauty.com
    http://www.luxury4him.com
6. **J Beverly Hills Rescue Anti-Aging Shampoo**
    http://www.haircareandbeauty.com
7. **Desert Essence Red Grape Shampoo**
    http://www.veganessentials.com
8. **Propoline Shampoo**
    http://www.apivita.com
9. **Avalon Organics Olive Oil and Grape Seed Moisturizing Shampoo**
    http://www.healthsuperstore.com
    http://www.vitacost.com
10. **Capilo Grape Seed Extract Shampoo**
    http://www.beautyofnewyork.com
11. **The Grape Seed Company Vine Therapy Shampoo**
    http://www.thegrapeseedcompany.com

NATURAL HAIR LOSS INGREDIENTS GROUP H-I

HEMP OIL

Hemp oil is the wondrous ingredient pressed from the hemp nut. Wondrous for the fact that it probably contains more essential fatty acids than any source researchers have found to date. These essential acids are fats necessary to the human body but unfortunately we cannot manufacture them ourselves. In particular this plant contains most of the polyunsaturated acids. Add to this the Omegas, linoleic acid, gamma linolenic acid, and a wealth of vitamins plus minerals and you have quite a list indeed.

Long confused with the extracts of the marijuana plant, hemp oil is a distinct product that has long been used by the American Indian and various cultures throughout the world.

Hemp oil when utilized in hair care and skin products does seem to have the remarkable quality of retarding the aging process. It is able to accomplish this feat because of a low molecular weight that allows a ready absorption into hair follicles and skin cells. This penetrating capacity leaves the skin and hair soft and pliant. This supplementation also allows our outer sheath to withstand harsh chemical treatments and climatic factors that it normally would not be able to. Because of this peculiar richness, in the fatty acids, hemp oil shampoos and conditioners should not be ignored as potential hair growth agents and baldness preventatives.

SOURCES FOR HEMP OIL

1. **Jason Hemp Enriched Shampoo**
   http://www.jasoncosmetics.com
2. **Hempz Shampoo and Conditioner**
   http://www.beautybrands.com
3. **Naturelle Hemp Shampoo**
   http://www.beautybasicsupply.com
   http://www.mikesbeautysupply.com
4. **Capillus Shampoos and Treatments**
   http://www.cannabis-cosmetics.com
5. **Natures Gate Hemp Nourishing Shampoo and Conditioner**
   http://www.natures-gate.com
   http://www.luckyvitamin.com
   http://www.vitacost.com
6. **Alterna Hemp Seed Shampoos and Conditioners**
   http://www.fashionandbeautystore.com
   http://www.haircareusa.com
7. **Azida Hemp Oil Shampoo and Conditioner**
   http://www.veganessentials.com
   http://www.azida.com

HEXANE

This lesser known chemical is used for a variety of purposes. The typical individual's exposure to it will be found as an anti-fungicidal in the treatment of dandruff, seborrhea, and psoriasis. It is also used in some of the newer hair care products as a deep pore-cleansing compound. Similar in purpose to the active ingredient ketoconazole, in Nizoral shampoo, appropriate claims of hair growth have surfaced with this ingredient.

In actual usage hexane can reduce the occurrence of the fungus pitysporum on the scalp. For years debate has surrounded what elimination of this fungus would do in regard to various afflictions of the skin and scalp. Current research that was dismissed for years tends to indicate a greater therapeutic value in controlling this fungus that once was thought. Even though other high-grade surfactants are able to reduce this fungus, elimination of it seems superior with chemicals such as hexane.

Interest seems to have grown for the fact that newer studies have shown hair growth may be activated by processes taking place in the upper portion of the hair follicle. In other words, investigations indicate this trigger mechanism may be more controllable than once thought. It is quite possible that some of these anti-fungicidals may activate the on/off switch for hair growth scientists have long been looking for. Regardless of this, these chemicals do have an anti-androgen effect, which reduces the formation of 5-alpha reductase on the scalp.

To increase this chemical's effectiveness some people have reported excellent results when combining with a biotin shampoo. To do this, first use a biotin shampoo. Rinse. Then apply the hexane-based product afterwards. Hair loss should decrease substantially if used at least once a week. Flaking and scaling should also dissipate.

- **These products can be left on the scalp for prolonged periods of time to increase their effectiveness. It will not harm the hair or scalp. These are deep pore cleansing compounds.**

PRODUCTS CONTAINING HEXANE

1. **Hask MD Medicated Shampoo**

2.   **Nioxin**

HONEY

One of the more overlooked ingredients for hair loss is honey. Early Egyptian pharaohs fearing thinning hair was a sign of disfavor among their various gods often utilized various formulations of honey to prevent hair loss. Still today many of the finest hair loss and hair care products utilize this ingredient both as growth agent and for a more luxurious and softer appeal to the tresses.

What makes honey so special? Well actually quite a few things make it so. First of all it's classified as a hygroscopic, which means it absorbs moisture from the surrounding air. Similar to humectants this ability to absorb water keeps the hair shaft soft and subtle decreasing breakage. Also by placing this ingredient into cosmetics and various scalp preparations this water retention ability helps rebuild the natural collagen levels deeper within the skin all necessary for youthful skin and hair growth.

Secondly since honey has natural anti-bacterial and anti-fungicidal properties it reduces inflammation on the scalp. As Israeli scientists demonstrated, in controlled studies, this reduction of various resistant bacteria allowed for the clearance of scalp seborrhea that had plagued some patients for years. In effect hair loss related to this condition was almost completely eliminated. This certainly leads to the question whether the hair loss was directly related to the condition or whether honey itself acted as a barrier to certain fungi or bacteria that are related to hair loss. Plus if you're wondering about every type of honey has proven to be beneficial in such cases but the darker brands have the highest degree of anti-oxidants.

- **A typical honey hair rinse can be made by mixing a spoon of honey into four cups of warm water. Add lemon juice if you are a blond.**

HONEY SOURCES

1.   **Beecolgy Honey & Botanical Sulfate-Free Shampoo http://www.beautysage.com**
2.   **Herbal Essences Honey Shampoo**
3.   **TIGI Catwalk Oatmeal & Honey Shampoo**

4. **Glossy Locks Honey and Coconut Milk Shampoo**
   http://www.100percentpure.com
5. **Manuka Honey**
   http://www.hollandandbarrett.com
   http://www.calcompnutrition.com

HYALURANONIC ACID

One substance you don't hear too much about is Hyluranonic acid. This constituent of many hair care products is one the many remarkable humectants. As you might remember humectants have the ability to draw moisture to the hair follicles and stimulate the minute nerves and blood vessels in the scalp. The one extremely big plus of this compound being that testing has indicated it to be a very effective dihydrotestosterone (DHT) inhibitor. These studies indicate that when massaged into the scalp via shampoo or conditioner this acid apparently blocks androgenic action that is a causative factor in hair loss. More study is needed though before the most suitable quantities, required for ideal results, can be determined.

- **Two of the most popular European hair loss treatments utilize hyluranonic acid, mucopolysaccharides, and saw palmetto, in their formulations. Their approximate cost is $1200 a year.**

- **We predict Hyluranonic acid may become one of the most popular ingredients for combating hair loss in the near future. It is a very potent DHT inhibitor with no notable side effects, when applied externally. Large American manufacturers have taken notice of this.**

SOURCES FOR HYALURANONIC ACID

1. **Episilk Shampoo with Pure Hyaluronic Acid**
   http://www.hyalogic.com
   http://www.vitamindeal.com
   http://www.911healthshop.com
2. **MD Strong Hyaluronic Acid & Aloe Moisture Shampoo**
   http://www.iwantthathair.com
3. **Nutra-Lift Healthy Hair Healthy Scalp Shampoo**
   http://www.nutra-lift.com

4. **Lamas Chinese Herbs Stimulating Shampoo**
    http://www.lamasbeauty.com
5. **Alterna Life Solutions and 10 Hair Care**
    http://www.haircareusa.com
    http://haircare.apothica.com
    http://www.beauty.com
    http://www.orderbeauty.com
    http://www.skinstore.com
6. **Biomedic Formula 1500 Intensive Therapy**
    http://www.hairwizards.com
7. **Progaine Shampoo**
8. **John Masters Organics Honey & Hibiscus Hair Reconstructing Shampoo**
    http://johnmasters.com

NATURAL HAIR LOSS INGREDIENTS GROUP J

JOJOBA OIL

Jojoba has been used since the day of the early American Indians. It is an excellent scalp cleanser and gives hair a thicker appearance. This cleansing ability comes from the low molecular weight of the oil that allows it to penetrate deeply into the pores of the scalp. Jojoba's composition is very similar to that of sebum in the skin. Rated as one of the better antioxidants it gives hair and skins a soft and pliant feel. The hair's natural sheen is also substantially increased. In addition to this, use of this lubricant can decrease hair breakage and brittleness considerably. Rancidity of the scalp is also diminished.

PRODUCTS CONTAINING JOJOBA OIL

1. **Joico BioJoba Shampoo**
2. **Nexus Biotin Shampoo**
3. **GNC Jojoba Shampoo and Conditioner (General Nutrition Stores)**
4. **Hobe Labs Super Hair Energizer with Jojoba Oil**
    http://www.houseofnutrition.com
    http://www.onlyhairloss.com
5. **Nexus Cysteine Shampoo**
6. **Hobe Labs Classic Hair Lover's Shampoo**
    http://hobelabs.com
7. **Jason Naturals Jojoba Shampoo and Conditioner**

8. **Mill Creek Jojoba Shampoo and Conditioner**
   http://www.webvitamins.com
9. **Nature's Gate Jojoba Shampoo**
   http://www.herbtrader.com
   http://www.vitaminshoppe.com
   http://www.swansonvitamins.com
10. **JR Liggetts Bar Shampoo Jojoba Peppermint Old-Fashioned**
    http://www.supplementwarehouse.com
11. **Focus 21 Jojoba Shampoo**
    http://www.haircareusa.com

JUICING

A phenomenon of the nineties that many people swear by is juicing. Juicing utilizes housewares appliances that extract the raw content of fruits and vegetables. According to juicers the ultimate way to derive the proper amount of vitamins, minerals, and carbohydrates necessary for the optimal performance of our body's systems, are through the juices. The body according to juicers cannot absorb supplements in tablet form to the degree it does with natural juices. As an example, a cup of strawberry juice containing 10,000 mg. of vitamin C would be readily absorbed by the body with little chance of side effects. Whereas, twenty 500 mg. tablets (10,000 mg) of vitamin C could easily result in a severe case of diarrhea and quite possibly a trip to the emergency room.

Also plants, vegetables, and fruits contain many more vitamins as compared to single supplements. This being the case, by juicing and combining the contents of these fruits and vegetables one could conceivably register greater savings. Since multiple vitamins are composed of synthetics and often inferior versions of many nutrients, to make them more affordable, what's bad for you may not be culled out.

Juicers also point out that trace minerals, fiber, amino acids, and components of the plants necessary for absorption in the body are also absent in most over the counter vitamins.

In relation to hair loss and baldness, juicers prescribe the juices of carrots and cucumbers to prevent hair loss. These can also be combined with red bell peppers, lettuce, spinach, and broccoli.

Accordingly, juicers claim that these vegetables supply the components of chromium, vanadium, and other trace minerals that cause baldness. Since over the counter vegetable products often use boiling, preservatives, and additives you often lose these minerals in the process.

Undoubtedly quite a few claims of juicers are backed by scientific evidence. Juicing is an ideal method for increasing nutrient absorption within the human body. Food processing does destroy many essential components of all foods. The convenience of these methods though is entirely up to the individual.

One very popular formula recommended for hair loss by Jay Kordich the "King of Juicers" is the following:
Five to Six Carrots
Handful of Alfalfa Sprouts
Four Lettuce Leafs

Combine all ingredients and juice. The alfalfa sprouts can be wrapped in the lettuce leafs.

- **Still today many people maintain that cucumbers are one of the better ingredients for combating hair loss. Substantial empirical research though has never been undertaken to validate this claim.**

<u>JUICING MACHINES</u>

1. **Various machines can be found in local department stores and through TV commercials.**
2. **Vegetable and juice products at your local grocer or nutritional stores.**
3. **Walmart Stores**

<u>**NATURAL HAIR LOSS SOLUTIONS GROUP K**</u>

<u>**KETOCONAZOLE-NIZORAL SHAMPOO**</u>

Nizoral is a product produced by Janssen Pharmaceutica. Its active ingredient is ketoconazole, an anti-fungicidal. It was developed for the treatment of dandruff, psoriasis, eczema, and various forms of dermatitis. The theory behind the product is that the fungus pitysporum is linked to many of these conditions. Janssen's research indicates that eliminating this fungus can eradicate these scalp and skin conditions. It is a prescription drug.

In regard to hair loss ketoconazole does have anti-androgen effects when used on the scalp. Since the shampoo has excellent deep cleansing abilities excess DHT is also eliminated. Many people do claim Nizoral stimulates hair growth and halts hair loss. Interestingly enough the actual hair growth could be related to improving the scalp's health and vitality to produce new hair follicles.

Ketoconazole the medication is present in the shampoo. By leaving the shampoo on the scalp for extended periods of time, before rinsing, you receive the maximum benefit of the medicine. It will not harm the hair. There is a cream formulation for other parts of the anatomy but it is more expensive. The cream though has been shown to be beneficial for a receding hairline. Because the product is highly concentrated many people are able to use a bottle for four to six months at a time. Suggested use patterns for Nizoral are only twice a week for a month and once a week thereafter. Following this anti-androgen routine many people have found this to be an excellent product for eliminating hair loss. Most doctors will readily write an unlimited prescription for the shampoo formula. Its retail price varies from ten to twenty dollars.

- **Sales of Nizoral seem to be escalating as reports of its ability to halt hair loss and increase hair growth increase. Besides being a very good shampoo it possesses a nice fragrance.**

- **Nizoral is now available without a prescription in a 1% concentration at most stores. It should be used twice a week for best results. Newer studies show it is as effective as the 2% version.**

- **Nizoral Cream left on the scalp for extended periods of time has shown itself to be an excellent treatment for the frontal hairline.**

- **Japanese researchers have reported astounding hair growth results when utilizing ketoconazole foam on the scalp for extended periods of time. The foam can be applied after shampooing with any shampoo. Preferably**

this should be done in the morning right after cleansing the scalp.

SOURCES FOR KETOCONAZOLE-NIZORAL SHAMPOO

1. **Doctor's prescription for 2% Nizoral Shampoo.**
2. **2% Ketoconazole Cream**
   http://www.northwestpharmacy.com
   http://www.canadianpharmacymeds.com
3. **Extina 2% Ketoconazole Foam**
4. **Hair Restoration Clinics**
5. **CVS Drug Stores - OTC 1% Nizoral**
6. **Walmart Stores - OTC 1% Nizoral**
7. **Canada Pharmacy**
   http://www.canadapharmacy.com/index.cfm
8. **Walgreens - OTC 1% Nizoral Shampoo**
9. **Regenepure DR**
   http://www.regenepure.com

NATURAL HAIR LOSS INGREDIENTS GROUP L

L-CARNITINE

Five small studies have substantiated that use of L-Carnitine either in supplemental form or applied topically can deter hair loss and stimulate new hair growth. So far though there is not a significant amount of anecdotal evidence to say one way or the other but what has been said is very positive. To tell you more about this supplement it is made within the human body from the amino acids lysine and methionine. It predominantly aids in fat metabolism and the normal growth and development of the body. It may aid in proper functioning of the kidneys and liver which are well known precepts of Chinese medicine for conquering hair loss. In natural form it can be found in avocados, milk, dairy products, and red meats such as beef and lamb.

Much of the popularity of this supplement grew from usage by "weight lifters" who label it as fat burner and energy producer. In other words this compound is capable of breaking down long chain fatty acids such as triglycerides to produce energy.

In respect to its ability to slow thinning hair and grow new hair we wholly endorse its topical use. This is an ingredient that seems to work its best when applied topically.

SOURCES FOR L-CARNITINE

1. **Hewley L-Carnitine Shampoo**
   http://www.hewley.com
2. **Vitacel 9**
   http://www.cellhealthmakeover.com
3. **Revita Shampoo**
   http://www.vitaminshoppe.com
   http://www.revitashampoostore.com
4. **Activ-M Shampoo and Leave In Lotion**
5. **Schwarzkopf 3D Shampoo**

LEMONGRASS

Lemongrass is a herb long associated with naturally derived "DHT blockers" and hair growth enhancement. Common to Southeast Asia it has long been utilized as a cooking ingredient in Thai food preparation. It possesses a quite pleasing fragrance and pleasant taste.

The herb itself has a multitude of uses ranging from an antiseptic to an anti-fungicidal. Studies at the University of Wisconsin showed that when 140 mg. capsules of lemongrass were used daily, significant reductions in cholesterol were produced. This may establish why DHT reduction did take place and why the oils of this herb may induce hair growth when applied to the scalp.

- **Lemongrass Oil can be added to the shampoo you are already using. Add about ¼ ounce per 8 ounces of shampoo.**

SOURCES FOR LEMONGRASS

1. **Label M Organic Moisturizing Lemongrass Shampoo**
   http://www.uniquelooks.com
2. **Nature's Gate, Organic Shampoo Lemongrass & Clary Sage**
   http://www.amerilifevitamin.com
3. **Mop Lemongrass Shampoo**
   http://www.beautybrands.com
   http://www.sleekhair.com

4. **Tigi Bed Head for Men - Clean Up Daily Shampoo**
   http://www.fragrancenet.com
5. **Health and Nutrition Stores**

LICORICE EXTRACT

Licorice is probably one of the most biologically active herbs in use today. To the Chinese only ginseng is viewed on a grander scale than this herb. The predominant active ingredient in this extract being glycyrrhetinic acid (GLA). Licorice has been shown to be effective in treating ulcers, skin problems, baldness, liver ailments, asthma, arthritis, and hypoglycemia. GLA has often been compared to hydrocortisone because of its anti-inflammatory actions.

In regard to hair loss apparently GLA has the ability to inhibit the conversion of testosterone to dihydrotestosterone (DHT), which is no small wonder since DHT is linked to hair fallout. Capsule and tea formulations are available for ingestion. Some people add the extract to shampoos and conditioners to achieve identical results. Herbal hair care products can be found with licorice extract included in them at nutrition stores.

- **Individuals with cardiac and kidney problems as well as those diagnosed with hypertension should avoid this herb.**

SOURCES FOR LICORICE EXTRACT

1. **Licorice is widely available and can be found at health and nutrition stores.**
2. **Walmart Stores.**
3. **Licorice Soaps**
4. **Philosophy Black Licorice High Foaming Shampoo, Shower Gel & Bubble Bath**
   http://www.totalbeauty.com
5. **Beija Flor Natural Licorice Root Extracts Elixir**
   http://beijaflornaturals.com
6. **Philou Licorice Shampoo**
   http://mp.hairboutique.com
7. **Korres Liquorice & Urtica Shampoo**
   http://www.bathandunwind.com

LINIMENT

One ingredient that has long been a component of hair loss preparations in China is liniment. Most liniments either contain camphor, oil of turpentine, oil of wintergreen, or ethyl alcohol. These liquids are often used by veterinarians to relieve pain by increasing circulation to an affected area. Herbalists claim that liniment applied to the scalp can stimulate blood flow enough to rekindle dormant hair follicles. No conclusive scientific research has ever truly established if this works are not. Chinese formulations often contain a "mixed bag" of additives when employing liniment. This is for dilution purposes and to nourish the hair follicles.

Since liniment can be a harsh product selective and careful usage is cautioned. Care should be taken when applying any product near the eyes. Application can produce temporary redness of the skin and a burning sensation. Liniment should be diluted with water or rubbing alcohol before using. Once done, apply sparingly with a washcloth.

- **There are several well-known brands of liniment found in stores that carry an extensive supply of alcohols, peroxides, glycerins, or topical treatments for the skin.**

SOURCES FOR LINIMENT

1. **Tiger Balm Liniment**
   http://www.drvita.com
2. **Kuz Hair Loss Control Cream and Shampoo**
   http://www.beautyofnewyork.com
   http://bluebeez.com

LUPEOL

Lupeol, a triterpene compound found in many plants, has received most of its exposure as an anti-cancer agent that could be capable of halting the spread of pancreatic cancer. At low concentrations, it has a remarkable ability to inhibit the synthesis of the testosterone receptor and to induce the expression of the FAS killing pathway in prostate cancer cells. In most cases there is nothing particularly fascinating about this because most natural substances require an abundance of the ingredient to eradicate cancer tumors which stifles their future use. This is not the case with lupeol because it is biologically active even at some of the lowest dosages. Lupeol is found in many fruits, vegetables, and herbs. This includes olives, strawberries, mangos, and figs.

In relation to hair loss many leading health experts have long maintained that the juices of strawberries and mangoes are particularly helpful in combating thinning hair because of the presence of Lupeol. This is particularly applicable to the mango.

SOURCES FOR LUPEOL

1.   **Fruit and Juice Section of Local Supermarkets and Health Stores.**

LYCOPENE

Lycopene is not traditionally thought of as a hair loss preventative or hair growth stimulant but newer research is beginning to show just the opposite. When recent studies were conducted with Lycopene it was found as effective as Proscar and Avodart in the treatment of BPH (benign prostatic hyperplasia). As many know this condition may be a precursor to cancer of this gland. Furthermore this antioxidant decreased the PSA levels and also inhibited the production 5 alpha reductase similar to what these popular prostrate and hair loss drugs do. What's a boon about this is it is a cheap all natural ingredient that both men and women can use without any risk of side effects. The caveat was it did not act as quickly for hair loss, as the mentioned, but similar results were seen over a course of time.

To expound more on these carotenoids they are what give the distinct red appearance to watermelon, pink grapefruit, and tomatoes plus the orange color seen in carrots. In the human body it is chiefly found in the fatty tissues and aids in vitamin A absorption. It does have a much more potent task than acting as a food coloring though. Lycopene has been shown to dramatically enhance the workings of the immune and cardiovascular systems. In fact large scale studies have shown that consumption of this antioxidant twice a week can reduce the incidence of heart disease by 50% or prostrate troubles by at least 30%.

If you want to use this vitamin it can be found in the mentioned fruits and vegetables, many prostate formulas, in multi-vitamins, or purchased as a stand-a-lone product. In regard to prostate formulas

Lycopene seems to work best with saw palmetto.

SOURCES FOR LYCOPENE

1. **The Vitamin Shoppe**
   http://www.vitaminshoppe.com
2. **Jarrow Prostate Optimizer**
   http://www.walgreens.com
3. **Urinozinc Prostate Wellness found at Walmart.**

LYSINE AND TAURINE

Two amino acids that have shown great promise in halting hair loss and promoting hair growth are Lysine and Taurine. The former also showing attention-grabbing results related to heart disease.

To elaborate on each of the two we will start with Lysine. Lysine like most of the amino acids can only be obtained from food sources or supplementation. It is necessary for processing fatty acids within the body, allowing the body to absorb calcium, and promotes the formation of collagen within the body. If you are a vegetarian you definitely might be deficient in this amino acid because plants do not contain this amino acid. Lysine for years has been used to combat herpes simplex and cold sores occurring in and around the mouth.

Studies involving the administration of L-Lysine have revealed remarkable scalp hair growth in those experiencing hair loss. A few British firms have shown that just the simple addition of L-Lysine supplements enhances the effects of minoxidil dramatically. It can be ingested in 500-1500 mg dosages one to three times a day, when using 2 or 5 percent minoxidil.

Taurine on the other hand is also an amino acid, but a tough one to locate in products. It like Lysine is only obtainable through the foods we eat or by supplementation. Taurine helps stabilize the excitability of cell membranes, which is of importance in the control of epileptic seizures. Taurine and sulfur are considered factors necessary for the control of the aging process and necessary for hair growth and the prevention of premature hair loss. Taurine also helps eliminate free radical wastes within the cells of our bodies.

- **Newer studies have shown that women experiencing**

unexplained hair loss may actually have both iron and lysine deficiencies. So before you make a trip to the doctor you might try these supplements.

• **With thyroid related hair loss you may exhibit a lysine deficiency.**

• **The latest research shows the results from minoxidil and Propecia are greatly enhanced with the use of lysine.**

SOURCES FOR LYSINE AND TAURINE

1. **Walmart Stores**
2. **GNC Stores**
3. **Walgreens**
4. **Folicure Conditioner**
   http://www.hairproducts.com
   http://www.beautyofnewyork.com
   http://sn2000.com
   http://www.sallybeauty.com
5. **Nioxin Intensive Therapy Clean Control**
6. **Schwarzkopf Activ-M Shampoo and Leave In Lotion**
   http://www.pakcosmetics.com
7. **Nutra Bio**
   http://nutrabio.com
8. **Supplements To Go**
   http://www.supplementstogo.com
9. **Seskavel Anti-Hair Loss Lotion, Shampoo, and Capsules**
   http://www.sesderma.com/usa/index.php
   http://www.skinelements.com
   http://aestheticsupplyonline.com

NATURAL HAIR LOSS INGREDIENTS GROUP M

MAGNESIUM OIL

One of the more notable aspects of pattern baldness is the increases in calcification within the follicle. Conversely this process is less present in those who don't experience the condition. Peculiarly this thickening is seen less often in women. Some scientists argue this increased calcification goes hand in hand with inflammation thereby being a major instigator of androgenetic alopecia. Research by Frederick Hoelzel in 1941 documented this relationship while removing the brains from 80 cadavers. It became fairly obvious to Hoelzel that cadavers with full heads of hair had experienced no calcification where in balding subjects this hardening of the skull bones was very much present. From this grew theories that if this calcification was reversed male pattern baldness could be substantially reduced. As time passed and more was learned about the human body quite a few scientists begin to suggest that various agents, such as magnesium oil and vitamins D-3 plus K-2, were quite capable of reducing this process.

The hypotheses behind the usage of these ingredients were to reduce the calcium found in soft issue, such as the scalp, and return it the bones and teeth where it should be. In turn androgenetic alopecia could be substantially retarded. Many leading researchers today still maintain that this inflammation process which attracts calcification is the key answer to baldness. Cure the inflammation within the follicle and the hair will grow once again.

If you want to test magnesium oil as a hair growth solution please remember to secure the purest form available. This mineral oil should not be used on recently injured skin or where the person is experiencing serious medical conditions. Other than that the oil is freely absorbed by the skin and excreted through the kidneys. The other caveat is magnesium oil can cause itching so it's wise to dilute it with water when necessary.

SOURCES FOR MAGNESIUM OIL

1. **Korres Magnesium and Wheat Proteins Toning Shampoo**
   http://www.skinsible.com
   http://www.bathandunwind.com
2. **Prehistoric Magnesium Oil**
   http://www.puremagoil.com
3. **Swanson Ultra Magnesium Oil**
   http://www.puremagoil.com
4. **DermaMag**
   http://www.magnesiumdirect.com
5. **Ancient Minerals Magnesium Oil**
   http://www.ancient-minerals.com

MAGNET THERAPY

Magnet therapy has its basis in effecting the meridians of the body similar to acupuncture in Chinese medicine. Touted as a low cost, non-addictive, and natural cure for many medical conditions, their use has grown substantially. In simplified terms magnets help the body regain its natural electromagnetic frequency.

Interestingly advocates of magnet therapy argue that since man is constantly exposed to the geo-magnetic effects of gravity his whole life is influenced by this magnetism. This magnetism in effect is fundamental to the cell renewal process of the human body. Proponents also argue that the energy that flows throughout the body is channeled through meridians very similar to a natural electro-magnetic field. It is only when these fields are disturbed or shielded from us is do we suffer from the ills that will follow. Magnets basically correct the imbalances associated with tissue damage and inflammation which cause pain and muscles to spasm.

Magnet therapy can act on nerve and muscle cells to relieve pain, relax tense muscles, and improve the circulation. As a cure for hair loss therapists suggest using flexible magnetic strips embedded in caps to stimulate blood flow. Though there is no scientific evidence to why, magnets in theory set up a vibration that enhances the blood flow in the minute capillaries of the scalp. By doing this dormant hair follicles are revived. The only caveat here is being that if you utilize a pacemaker for the heart it is not advisable to try this.

- **Magnetic Therapy may be covered as an alternative treatment under some health insurance policies.**

SOURCES FOR MAGNET THERAPY

1. **Mag Gro**
   http://www.onlyhairloss.com
2. **Magnetic Hair Brush**
   http://www.magnetictherapymagnets.com/magneticbrush.html
   http://www.discovermagnetics.com/dm_magnetic_brush.html
   http://www.lhasaoms.com
   http://www.folica.com

MANGANESE

The word manganese is derived from the Greek word for magic and without a doubt the term is well deserved. This mineral is one of the building blocks for healthy bones, hair, and nails in our bodies. This unique substance makes up part of the molecules known as mucopolysaccharides in our body. These saccharide compounds are an absolute essential for the development and continued health of hair follicles on the scalp. Research indicates that a deficiency of this trace mineral may be growing in Western cultures. The reasoning behind this is that the proliferation of processed and frozen foods has led to a deficit of whole grains in the diet.

Since manganese is a trace mineral in our diet, individuals are cautioned not to overuse it. Proper amounts of this nutrient can be found in most multi-vitamins.

SOURCES FOR MANGANESE

1. **Found in most complete OTC multi-vitamins.**
2. **Centrum Multi-Vitamins**
3. **GNC Vitamins for the Hair**
4. **Nioxin**

MASSAGE

Swedish research and massage therapists have maintained for years that baldness is the result of the tightening of the underlying thin membrane of skin beneath the scalp. This area is appropriately named the crown galea or galea aponeurotica. This tightening increases as we age and during the thinning process associated with hair loss. As evidence of this advocates of this theory point to the loss of flexibility and evaporation of fat deposits in the scalp associated with male pattern baldness. To witness this one can place fingers on the head and use a back and forth rocking motion to flex the skin. If the areas show little movement blood flow has probably decreased to the tightened areas. Likewise transplant specialists often use a similar test to see if recipient sites will have enough blood supply for the donor plugs.

To massage the scalp one should place the palms of the hand on the sides of the head while the fingertips work the upper scalp in an unhurried circular fashion. This should produce redness in the areas where the blood flow is stimulated. Try to avoid vigorous motion since this can lead to breakage of the hair. An ideal time to do this is after showering while in front of a mirror. This allows you to view the areas that are being stimulated. These scalp manipulations allow the pores to open for increased absorption. This is ideal when application of hair treatments is desirable.

SOURCES FOR MASSAGE EQUIPMENT

1. **Nism Massaging Hair Brush**
   http://www.herbalremedies.com
2. **The Cosmetic Center Stores**
3. **Brainwave Scalp Stimulator**
   http://www.ebodylogic.com
   http://www.walkinbackrub.co.uk
4. **Your local hair stylist.**
5. **K-Mart**
6. **Walmart**
7. **The Crown Scalp Stimulator**
   http://webhome.idirect.com/~rivela1
8. **Scalp Stimulator**
   http://www.folliclestimulator.com
9. **Shape Your Face**
   http://www.shapeyourface.com

MELATONIN TOPICAL

Melatonin's chief source of fame is as an OTC supplement for insomnia. It is a derivative of the amino acid tryptophan. In theory it regulates the sleep-wake cycles of the brain otherwise known as circadian rhythms. In practice this supplement has proved to be highly effective in treating minor sleep disorders and jet lag. The caveat being here is that with any type drug which induces sleep the body can rapidly become dependent on it. Also melatonin has been shown to further agitate depression in some people. What's most notable about melatonin though is it probably one of the most effective free radical scavengers among all vitamins and herbs. But the caution again is that it docs induce sleep so its benefits would be limited. Topical solutions of melatonin have been around for a while chiefly as a sunscreen when combined with vitamin A and C plus aloe.

Anecdotal evidence of the topical use of melatonin for hair growth has been recorded but not until recently has it been established scientifically. In a small German study of women treated with topically applied melatonin, for six months, there was a definitive increase of hair follicles in the growth phase. The subjects were experiencing the established symptoms of genetic female pattern baldness. Conclusions of the study were that melatonin was effective in treating genetic hair loss especially of the frontal hairline.

Our suggestion based upon the anecdotal reports about melatonin is that topical formulas might prove very effective for males and females who are experiencing frontal hair loss. Since topical formulas can be purchased cheaply it could prove to be an effective weapon against pattern baldness. There are no recorded side effects with the use of topical melatonin.

SOURCES FOR MELATONIN TOPICAL

1. **Life-Flo Melatonin Cream**
   http://www.foodsofnature.com
   http://www.vitasprings.com
   http://www.vitacart.com
   http://www.energeticnutrition.com
2. **Hair Again**
   http://youngagain.com
3. **Allvia Integrated Melatonin**
   http://www.ovitaminpro.com
4. **Asatex – Swiss product with limited availability.**
5. **Oral Melatonin**
   http://www.vitaminshoppe.com
   http://www.walgreens.com
   http://www.gnc.com

MENTHOL AND EUCALYPTUS

These botanicals when applied act as vasodilators. This effect increases the circulation in blood vessels by temporally widening them. You will see and feel a harmless tingling and reddening of the skin during use. Many people find this effect quite enjoyable. Menthol in addition can temporarily reduce itching when applied externally.

PRODUCTS CONTAINING MENTHOL AND EUCALYPTUS

1. **Denorex Tar Shampoo**
2. **John Frieda Root Awakening**
   http://www.johnfrieda.com
3. **Thicker Fuller Hair Shampoo and Conditioner –
   Found in shampoo section of many retail stores.**
4. **Biotene Shampoo**
5. **Vitalize Shampoo**
   http://www.escentsaromatherapy.com
6. **Groganics Daily Topical Scalp Treatment**
   http://www.webplusbeauty.com
7. **Prevent Hair Loss Treatment**
8. **Terax Bosco Revitalizing Shampoo**
   http://www.sleekhair.com
9. **Wildly Natural Seaweed Argan Shampoo: Eucalyptus
   & Peppermint Scent**
   http://www.seaweedbathco.com
10. **Lemon Eucalyptus Shampoo**
    http://www.keywestaloe.com

MSM - METHYLSULPHONYLMETHANE

MSM (Methylsulphonylmethane) is a substance you will gradually hear more and more about. The hype about this ingredient is tremendous. Some of it is deserved, some which is not. One thing research though has corroborated is that MSM does accelerate the growth rate of hair. Whether it prevents hair loss and promotes new hair growth has not been established empirically, but a large amount of anecdotal evidence seems to indicate it does.

MSM to elaborate is a naturally occurring organic sulfur compound found in about every form of unprocessed fresh food, especially fruits, milk, meat, seafood, and vegetables. The compound itself can be found in the tissues of all living organisms. Next to salt and water it is the third most common substance found in the human body. It is fundamental to the bodies' functions of cell repair and renewal, immune system functioning, and resistance to parasites and allergens. It is not a sulfate preservative or derivative.

So what's the hitch and why do you need it? The problem here is that even though many foods contain it, most of it is destroyed during food processing, cooking, or steaming. Plus your body cannot produce it so you must derive it from the food you consume or by supplementation. The catch here is that even though few people have known deficiencies the use of MSM seems to be a panacea for many ailments. Hair loss being one of them. Since the hair and nails utilize sulfur for growth it is understandable why an increase of this substance in the body could accelerate the developmental process.

As for safety concerns this supplement is basically harmless. If the body ingests too much, it just excretes it rather rapidly. Often times MSM is used by arthritis sufferers with Glucosamine.

- **The availability of MSM has increased substantially and it can now be found in most drug stores.**

SOURCES FOR MSM - METHYLSULPHONYLMETHANE

1. **TriMedica MSM Shampoo**
   http://www.herbalremedies.com
   http://www.evitamins.com
2. **Soignee Botanicals Shampoo and Conditioner**
   http://www.ocnaturals.com
   http://livesuperfoods.com
3. **Gaines Nutrition. Excellent source for MSM supplements.**
   http://www.gaines.com
4. **MSM Shampoo and Conditioner**
   http://www.herbalremedies.com/haircare.html
5. **Dr. Ron's MSM Shampoo and Conditioner**
   http://www.drrons.com/shampoos-conditioners.htm

MILK THISTLE

Milk thistle (Silybum Marinum) is a well-known herb used for the protection of the liver. It can be highly beneficial to anyone who consumes alcohol, smokes, takes drugs whether legal or illegal, or lives in areas with a high amount of pollution. The herb itself is often prescribed to reduce the symptoms of hepatitis, cirrhosis, and even mushroom poisoning. Chinese herbalists often prescribe milk thistle to combat hair loss. The reasoning behind this is these herbalists maintain pattern baldness is related to liver impairment. It is a common herb found in many vitamin sections of leading stores

SOURCES FOR MILK THISTLE

1.   **Spring Valley Herbs.**
2.   **The Vitamin Shoppe**
     http://www.vitaminshoppe.com
3.   **Folicure Conditioner**
4.   **Nature's Way Standardized Milk Thistle**
     http://www.swansonvitamins.com

MINOXIDIL

Minoxidil is currently one of the few FDA approved drugs for the treatment of baldness in the United States. The Upjohn Corporation owns the product's patent. Originally used as a heart medication called Loniten (minoxidil), the drug was observed to cause hirsutism (hair growth) when consumed orally. Subsequently clinical testing was undertaken to learn if minoxidil could yield hair growth in topically applied areas of the scalp. These studies led to approval of minoxidil, first as a prescription drug and later as an OTC drug.

As many people now know this product is marketed as Rogaine in the United States and Regaine outside of it. The product formulation is available in 2% and 5% strengths. The 2% and 5% formulas can be found in generic versions. The reason for this is the patent has expired on of these strengths. Both offerings are available on the Internet and retail stores.

Rogaine's greatest effectiveness has been shown in the crown portion of the scalp. Few results have been achieved in frontal areas of the scalp except with ointment or salve formulas. Formulations containing retonic acid (vitamin A) appear to show the greatest promise for dealing with receding hairlines. Currently many stores offer generic versions of Rogaine, which are of exactly the same quality as Upjohn's original product. The chief reason we report on minoxidil is that some of the generic versions now cost as little as $2.99 a bottle. Plus this product has been shown to have few if any side effects.

One way people have turned minoxidil into an effective an affordable treatment is by utilizing this method. Apply one dosage a day after shampooing on a daily or rotating day basis. The purpose of this is to strictly retard hair loss and continue stimulating the blood supply to areas that may recede. Quite a few people claim this method is probably the most affordable answer for stopping hair loss. In theory by purchasing 2% generic versions the cost would run about two to four dollars a month to extinguish hair loss. Quite the opposite of what you might think just one dosage a day seems to as effective as two in most cases. As progressively more research appears the true strength of minoxidil in 2% formulations may be in doing just as is suggested. We entirely endorse this solution as a workable and viable alternative. Stronger formulations of minoxidil (5%) can be used in a similar fashion.

- **A growing number of minoxidil users claim that it is an excellent aphrodisiac. Even though applied topically supposedly the active ingredients can still stimulate the sex drive of both men and women. No empirical research has substantiated these claims as yet.**

- **Generic versions of minoxidil or Rogaine are often produced by precisely the same companies. This is normally listed on the boxes. Often time's large third party companies are commissioned to produce products in quantity.**

- **With many hair loss treatments there may be a slight accretion in hair fallout upon initial use. This loss comes from hair in its telogen phase or shedding stage of hair growth. This increase is normal and does subside within a short period of time. Such occurrences are ordinary when first using a variety of drugs. It even occurs while switching among shampoos and conditioners that might be harsher than what you previously might have been using. So don't let it alarm you. It occurs all the time and you've probably just never realized it or had reason to observe it. These treatments do not affect healthy hair in the growth stage or anagen phase. Many authorities in this matter claim that this fallout is rewarding because similar to plucking hair it quickens the pace of returning hair to its growth stage. We don't recommend plucking your hair, though.**

- **Price drops can be expected yearly with Rogaine. The rationale seems to be that Upjohn is repositioning itself because of continued competition from Propecia.**

- Rogaine in the 5% formulation is oilier than the 2% version to increase its absorption into the hair follicles. Because of this scalp drying times are extended.

- Regrowth time may begin as early as two months with Extra Strength Rogaine. Some studies show this 5% formula is forty-six percent more effective. Plus the coverage is three times greater over a one year period, when compared with the 2% formula. Other researchers maintain the 2% strength will produce exactly the same results. It just takes a while longer, but it's cheaper.

- The makers of Rogaine provide auto-fill programs on their internet site for their Extra Strength Formula for Men and the Regular Strength Formula for Women. You can inquire about "no risk buyback" programs that allow you to experiment with the product. We always encourage asking your doctor for samples to see if it's the thing for you.

- Rogaine now claims even greater effectiveness with its new foam.

PRODUCTS CONTAINING MINOXIDIL

1. Equate 2% & 5% Minoxidil (Walmart Stores)
2. CVS 2% & 5% Minoxidil
3. Walgreens 2% & 5% Minoxidil
4. Costco 5% Kirkland Minoxidil (Excellent prices)
5. Polaris Labs NR-07 Hair Growth Treatment
   http://www.folica.com
   http://www.vitasprings.com
   http://polarisresearchlabs.com
6. Minoxidil Salve, Gel, and Ointment
   http://www.zooscape.com
7. Rogaine
8. Walgreens
9. Generic Minoxidil Foam
   http://www.minoxidildirect.com
   http://www.c-star.net
10. Kirkland Brand Generic Minoxidil
    Costco

http://www.salonweb.com/minoxidil
http://www.onlyhairloss.com
http://kirklandminoxidil.co.uk

MUCOPOLYSACCARIDES, TRICOSACCARIDES, AND OGLIOSACCARIDES

These unusual names belong to a group of ingredients developed by Crinos Industria Italia during the 1980's. They are known as humectants. Extensive testing as topical solutions for the treatment of baldness were conducted and are still being overseen by this company. Crinos Industria is recognized as a world leader in hair loss research.

Humectants, to elaborate, are molecules that pull liquids from the surrounding atmosphere to the skin. They can do so at ratios of one to one, or up to three hundred to one with some of the newer formulations and hydroxyl compounds. These ingredients quickly found their way into cosmetics for women to increase the fluid retention capabilities and youthful appearance of the skin. Even though scientists had known for years drinking your daily quota of liquids were highly beneficial to the body's outer sheath, they knew, maintaining this youthful radiance was best achievable by supplementing the skin. In this particular case with saccharide compounds that absorbed the water from the surrounding air. The whole purpose of this, as you might surmise, was to prevent premature wrinkling of the skin. Research at this time also began to show that this moisturizing effect was even more valuable to hair follicles on the scalp. Similar to vitamin A and D derivatives, you have heard so much about; these saccharide compounds seem to have a similar effect with regard to hair growth. By application in the desired area moisture is drawn to the hair follicle. This in turn strengthens and rejuvenates the small blood vessels in the dermis. By strengthening this network of capillaries the continued health of the follicle is assured.

What's truly ideal about the saccharide compounds is that because of their low molecular weight they could be readily absorbed into the follicles. Plus these agents were free of any sticky or greasy residue found in oils. As even more recent studies disclosed these compounds were astounding boons to increasing the longevity of hair follicles particularly in thinning areas of the scalp. At worse they decreased the early breakage and over-stretching of the hair shaft common to hair loss.

One other important thing to point out is that these ingredients have a vasodilator effect on the scalp. This is a condition where the small blood vessels in the application area are widened. Due to this you should observer a slight tingling or redness where applied. This is completely harmless and does not always occur.

- **The following products can be used on a daily basis and their affordability should allow you to do so. No particular schedule is necessary except in the case of Foltene or Folicure. Enclosed with these products are ampoules to be used on alternating days during the first six to eight weeks of your treatment program.**

- **These ingredients are labeled as Glycosaminoglycan's.**

- **Since water retention in the skin is one of the most effective ways to halt free radical damage, caused by the aging process, these constituents can prove highly beneficial to the hair follicle.**

PRODUCTS CONTAINING MUCOPOLYSACCARIDES, TRICOSACCARIDES, AND OGLIOSACCARIDES

1. **Focus 21 Sea Plasma Shampoo and Conditioner**
2. **Anthony Logistics Body Building Hair Thickening Shampoo**
   http://www.sephora.com
3. **Awaken & Replenish Shampoo**
   http://www.healthyhairplus.com
4. **Folicure Shampoo, Conditioner and Thinning Hair Treatment**
   http://www.sn2000.com
5. **Thicker Fuller Hair Care Products**
6. **Herbal Glo Thinning Hair Shampoo and Conditioner**
   http://www.hbees.com/herbalglo.html
   http://www.beautynaturally.com
   http://www.pennherb.com
7. **Rexsol Nixodil**
   http://www.rexsol.com
8. **Scruples Hair Care Products**
9. **KMS Shampoos**
10. **Joico Hair Care Products**

11. **Matrix Hair Care Products**
12. **Zotos International Thinning Hair System**
13. **Jason Thin To Thick Hair and Scalp Therapy System**
    http://www.jason-natural.com/
    http://www.swansonvitamins.com
    http://www.iherb.com

MUIRA PUAMA

Muira puama often described as the "potency wood" is a small tree native to the thickest rainforests of Brazil and dense jungles of Africa. As one might guess the reputation it earned came from centuries of use as an aphrodisiac and cure for erectile dysfunction. Both men and women use the herb. Whether this herbs quality is related to its ability to enhance physical or psychological well being has never been fully determined. There are also no known health risks associated with this herb.

Specifically muira puma contains what are referred to as long fatty acids, sterols, terpenes, alkaloids, tannins, essential oils, esters, and beta sitosterol.

Muira Puama's relationship to enhancing hair growth and hair loss prevention was chiefly exhibited in studies related to increasing sexual performance. The herbs numerous sterols have been linked with an ability to inhibit the conversion of testosterone to DHT. Many users of the herb did report a slowing of hair fallout and some hair growth.

We caution people in using this herb in combination with Yohimbe. Muira Puama is not associated with any health risks. Yohimbe on the other hand has been associated with many medical emergencies such as rapid heart beat, high blood pressure, panic attacks, dizziness, and headaches.

SOURCES FOR MUIRA PUAMA

1. **Green Bush Natural Products**
   http://www.greenbush.net/muirpuam1oun.html
2. **Solaray Muira Puama**
   http://www.houseofnutrition.com
   http://www.vitaminshoppe.com
3. **Physician Formulas Muira-Puama**

http://www.physicianformulas.com

NATURAL HAIR LOSS INGREDIENTS GROUP N

NA PCA OR SODIUM PCA

Sodium PCA is the skin's natural humectants. Its ability to draw moisture to the skin from the surrounding atmosphere makes it far superior to most man made oils. With aging our bodies produce less of this ingredient which results in hardening and wrinkling of the skin. Lesser known schools of thought believe that baldness has a link to the loss of this moisture in the scalp. Products containing Na PCA increase the hair's elasticity and give it a fuller appearance.

PRODUCTS CONTAINING NA PCA OR SODIUM PCA

1. **Focus 21 Sea Plasma Hair Care Products**
2. **Progaine Shampoo and Conditioner**
3. **Zincplex**
   http://www.zincplex.com
4. **A.G Hair Cosmetics**
   http://www.beautycarechoices.com
5. **Lanza Healing Pure Clarifying Shampoo**
   http://www.beautyclicks.com
6. **Beauty Without Cruelty Moisture Plus Shampoo**
   http://www.beautywithoutcruelty.com
7. **Twinlab Na-PCA**
   http://www.webvitamins.com
   http://www.ihealthtree.com
   http://www.iherb.com/

NANO SHAMPOO AND CONDITIONER

Nano Shampoo is a proprietary product developed by Doctor Peter Proctor of Houston, Texas. Proctor is a noted researcher in the area of hair loss. According to Dr. Proctor nitric oxides are the chemicals that turn on the switch for hair growth. Superoxide's produced by the immune cells, which accumulate around the hair follicles, turn off this switch according to his extensive research.

Quite a few people claim Nano Shampoo is one of the better products for halting hair loss and stimulating growth. Doctor Proctor's product line does include a conditioner. The primary ingredient is Pyridine N-Oxides. Claimed results are similar to minoxidil. A three month's supply of either product runs about $39.95. Since the product does have quite a following on the Internet we include it for consideration

- **With this product the medicine is in both the shampoo and conditioner. This being so, people often leave either product in the hair for extended periods of time before rinsing. Most people have found that a twice a week schedule of either product yields very good results. Using both products on the same day may be duplicative and costly.**

- **Doctor Proctor also produces another product for the treatment of baldness called Proxiphen. It is somewhat more expensive.**

- **One well-known international pharmaceutical company in the past year has filed numerous patents for compounds containing nitric oxides for the treatment of baldness.**

SOURCES FOR NANO SHAMPOO AND CONDITIONER

1. **Hair Loss 101**
   http://hairloss101.com
2. **Life Extension Index**
   http://www.lef.org/prod_desc/index.html
3. **Dr. Proctor's site**
   http://www.drproctor.com
4. **Only Hair Loss**
   http://www.onlyhairloss.com

NEEM OIL

The Neem tree (Azadirachta Indica) is a tropical evergreen related to the mahogany tree. Native to east India and Burma, it grows in much of Southeast Asia and West Africa. As demand for the oil of this tree has increased it has been transplanted to Caribbean and Central American countries. In locations where the temperature does not drop below fifty degrees the tree can grow as tall as 100 feet. The life span of the tree can easily run in excess of 200 years. Plus it requires little rainfall to flourish.

For centuries the people of India have revered the properties of Neem oil. Millions have used it to clean teeth, treat various skin disorders, and as a health tonic. The tree has relieved so many different pains, fevers, infections, and other complaints that it has been labeled "the village pharmacy" in many part of Asia.

Two decades of research have revealed promising results in so many disciplines that this obscure species may be of enormous benefit to countries both poor and rich. Even some of the most cautious researchers believe that indeed Neem deserves to be called a "wonder plant".

The Neem tree contains several thousand various chemicals. Of special interest are the terpenoids that are unique to Neem. The most active of these being azadirachitin.

In relation to hair loss Ayruvedic practitioners have long prescribed the neem oil as a hair loss preventative and regrowth agent. Though few studies have actually been conducted to substantiate this anecdotal evidence is abundant. If you desire to use this oil we suggest looking for shampoos and conditioners that contain it. The pure extract could be a little greasy.

SOURCES FOR NEEM OIL

1. **Theraneem Scalp Therape Shampoo**
    http://www.vitaminshoppe.com
    http://www.swansonvitamins.com
2. **Ecco Bella Holistic Remedies Green Tea and Neem Shampoo**
    http://www.eccobella.com
    http://www.luckyvitamin.com
    http://www.4allvitamins.com
3. **Better Botanicals Neem Care Shampoo**
    http://www.betterbotanicals.com
4. **Health and Nutrition Stores**
5. **100 Percent Pure Burdock & Neem Shampoo**
    http://www.100percentpure.com

NIACIN

Niacin is one of the many B-vitamins. It is also known as nicotinic acid. When used in enough quantity it produces a "flushing" of the skin due to the release of histamine in the body. This temporary reddening is also due to the stimulation of blood flow. As pointed out earlier this histamine release is a noted hair growth factor. This being the case niacin is often used with hair loss products to widen the pores for absorption and increase blood flow to the follicle. Niacin is frequently combined with biotin products. Along with being another antioxidant, this vitamin has a calming effect similar to Valium, in some people.

- **Niacin is probably one of the few nutrients recognized by the medical community as having the ability to reduce cholesterol. It is definitely one of the "spark plugs" that keeps skin and hair tissue healthy.**

- **The best way to find a niacin product is to look for one containing biotin. Biotin works best when combined with niacin.**

PRODUCTS CONTAINING NIACIN

1. **Grow Shampoo and Conditioner**
   http://www.hairformula37.com
2. **GNC Brands Biotin Products and Vitamins**
3. **Nexus Biotin Shampoo**
4. **Biotene Shampoo**
5. **Fine Solutions with Niaplex**
   http://www.cachebeauty.com/hair_loss.htm
6. **Revivogen Shampoo**
   http://www.onlyhairloss.com
7. **Regenepure NT Hair Regrowth Shampoo**
   http://www.regenepure.com
8. **Magick Botanicals Shampoo and Conditioner for Thinning Hair (scented and unscented formulas)**
   http://magickbotanicals.com
   http://www.greenmarket.com
9. **Nioxin Shampoos**

NIOXIN

A group of products we now include in their own category because of concentrated formulations and decreases in prices are those made by Nioxin. These products are scientifically developed with botanical agents, amino acids, proteins, vitamins, and DHT agents acting synergistically to combat thinning hair.

To elaborate more on Nioxin products they are for both men and women and include shampoo, conditioner, hair spray, and treatment formulations for dry, oily, normal, and chemically treated hair. Some of the treatment solutions designed specifically for areas of excessive hair loss and the frontal hairline are Hair Booster, Scalp Renew, and Diamax. They are truly unique products with active ingredients anyone faced with thinning hair should consider.

- **Nioxin has introduced its new systems approach for dealing with the various stages of thinning hair and hair loss. Since there are eight unique systems be sure to choose the one just right for you.**

SOURCES FOR NIOXIN

1. **Hair Care and Beauty Shops**
2. **Nioxin**
   http://www.nioxin.com
3. **VBS Beauty**
   http://vbsbeauty.com
4. **Discount Beauty**
   http://www.discount-beauty.com
5. **Hello Gorgeous**
   http://store.hello-gorgeous.net
6. **Beauty Clicks**
   http://www.beautyclicks.com
7. **Pandora Beauty**
   https://www.pandorabeauty.com
8. **Beauty Deals**
   http://www.beautydeals.net

NORWEGIAN KELP

Norwegian kelp (Ascophyllum Nodosum) is harvested every four years from the deep oceans surrounding the countries of Norway and Iceland. It's unique in that it is not prone to the pollutants seen with kelp derived from shallower waters. Also because it is harvested from colder subterranean waters its sheen is a deep brown as compared to the greener varieties you may be familiar with. Due to these peculiarities this form of kelp is also richer in iodine than the blue-green variety. It also contains twelve other vitamins, 60 minerals, and 20 amino acids, which facilitate many enzymatic processes within the body.

Many Scandinavian companies claim this unique form of kelp is the panacea for a broad range of hair loss problems.

SOURCES FOR NORWEGIAN KELP

1. **Zooscape**
    http://www.zooscape.com
2. **VitaNet Health Foods**
    http://vitanetonline.com
3. **Walmart Stores**
4. **Natural Food and Vitamin Shops**

NATURAL HAIR LOSS INGREDIENTS GROUP O

OLIVE OIL

The olive tree is an evergreen native to the Mediterranean regions but is widely grown in tropical areas and warm climates. Olive oil has been used effectively in many ways. First, its leaves are utilized as an antiseptic, astringent, febrifuge, and tranquilizer. Second its oils act as a chologue, demulcent, emollient, cooking ingredient, and a laxative. Thirdly as a hair care ingredient, fever reducer, and laxative. The most common usage though is a base for liniments and ointments.

Olive oil has probably been used more than anything else as an ingredient for stimulating hair growth. The reasoning probably relates to its ability to reduce cholesterol internally and externally. With alcohol it makes a good hair tonic and with rosemary a good treatment for dandruff. Even though no empirical research has ever been done to establish its hair growing qualities anecdotal evidence has persisted for years. The trick though is in finding products that use it as a primary ingredient. Olive oil soap can be used in much the same way as a shampoo. You'll be surprised at how soft it can leave your skin and hair.

SOURCES FOR OLIVE OIL

1. **Kiehl's Olive Fruit Oil Nourishing Shampoo**
   http://www.kiehls.com
2. **Cayce Cures**
   http://www.caycecures.com
   http://www.baar.com
3. **Health and Nutritional Stores**
4. **Regis Salons - Regis Design Line Olive Oil Shampoos and Conditioners**
5. **BioInfusion Olive Oil Shampoos and Conditioners**
6. **Frederic Fekkai Glossing Shampoo**
   http://www.planetbeauty.com
   http://www.fekkai.com

ORANGE AND GRAPE JUICE

Unusual as it might sound there are people who steadfastly maintain that orange and grape juice consumed daily can reduce your hair loss. As to what kind, fresh is preferable, but concentrate or frozen will do just fine. Other than the fact that these juices are high in potassium, niacin, vitamin C, and bioflavanoids, the basis for these claims seems a bit outrageous.

Promoters of this solution argue the best time to ingest these enjoyable beverages is before retiring. Accordingly the nutrients found in the juices are best absorbed at night for the self-healing of the body. This assimilation into your system is based upon considerable scientific evidence as to the ideal times for consumption of most medications, for rebuilding of the cellular system. These theories might be diametrical to what you might have previously been taught.

Since these juices are relatively inexpensive and next to water probably some of the better tasting, it certainly couldn't hurt to sample them. Amazingly it seems to work in some cases, but no medical research would indicate it should produce results.

SOURCES FOR ORANGE AND GRAPE JUICE

1. **All grocery stores**
2. **Vitamin and nutritional stores**

NATURAL HAIR LOSS INGREDIENTS GROUP P

PIROCTONE OLAMINE

Piroctone Olamine, often referred to Octopirox, is an anti-fungicidal often put to use in shampoos for the prevention of dandruff and seborrheic dermatitis. It is considered one of the least toxic of the many ingredients utilized for the treatment of these maladies. Like many of these fungicidal ingredients it has shown an ability to curb hair loss, increase the diameter of the present hair, and stimulate new hair growth. In comparative testing between zinc pyrithione, Nizoral, and Piroctone Olamine, the latter proved to be the most effective in preventing hair loss. Testing also showed that Piroctone Olamine based products had superior anti-androgenic properties that were useful in the delaying the onset of female and male pattern baldness if used on a regular basis. Many people will find this to be incredibly good news in Europe and Mexico but there tends to be a limited availability in the United States. Top brands such as Head and Shoulders employing zinc pyrithione have long entrenched themselves as the product of choice in North America.

SOURCES FOR PIROCTONE OLAMINE

1. **Folicure Dandruff Shampoo**
2. **SebaMed**
   http://www.feelunique.com
3. **SachaJuan Scalp Hair Shampoo**
   http://www.luxury4him.com
4. **Juniper Mint Scalp Therapy Shampoo**
   http://www.tonymaleedyhair.com
5. **Reistill Anti Hair Loss Shampoo**
6. **Eucerin Anti-Dandruff Shampoo**
   http://pharmamundi.com
7. **Sesderma Sebovalis Therapeutic Shampoo**
   http://pharmamundi.com
   http://bellapielstore.com

8. **Una Dandruff Shampoo**
   http://www.unahairproducts.com
9. **Sebenol Dandruff Shampoo**
   http://www.beautyofnewyork.com
10. **Australian Tea Tree Anti-Dandruff Shampoo**
    http://www.beautynaturals.com
    http://www.hawthornhealth.com
11. **Ginger Anti-Dandruff Shampoo**
    http://www.thebodyshop-usa.com
12. **Glytone by Ducray Elution Dermo-Protective Shampoo**

PREZATIDE COPPER

Loren Pickart a distinguished researcher at the University of California discovered that these compounds previously used to heal wounds were useful in the treatment of male pattern baldness. Later a researcher at the University of Wisconsin claimed, with his studies, that prezatide copper was twenty times more effective than minoxidil.

The formula itself is derived from a chain of three amino acids found in blood, urine, and saliva that bind with copper to stimulate the body's natural healing process. The most active ingredient biologically being prezatide copper.

Folligen the formulation developed by Pickart is a currently purchasable product. Its ingredients are on the safe and approved list of the FDA. A similar formulation of this product Tricomin has also received full FDA approval as a treatment for pattern baldness. Tricomin itself is expected to have widespread commercial availability. It is an over the counter product and a prescription will not be needed to obtain it.

One of the reasons we report on this compound is that many people have found it highly effective. The other reason being is that the typical contents of the product will normally last an individual about three months. This could vary dependent upon the area of the scalp being treated. Prezatide Copper has also been reported to be more effective on the frontal hairline than minoxidil. This being the case prezatide copper could be used to supplement the forward areas of the scalp. Minoxidil on the other hand could be used in the crown portions of the scalp, where it is documented as having its greatest effectiveness.

- **Prezatide Copper formulations should be applied at least three times a week before retiring.**

- **Tricomin products are available now. The hair loss lineup includes shampoos, conditioners, and treatment agents. These products are expensive.**

SOURCES FOR PREZATIDE COPPER

1. **Folligen**
    http://www.folica.com
    http://www.onlyhairloss.com
    http://store.reverseskinaging.com
2. **Tricomin**
    http://www.onlyhairloss.com
    http://www.tricomin.com
    http://www.skinstore.com
    http://www.drugstore.com

PROCAPIL

Procapil is one of the newer patented agents for combating hair loss. Basically this ingredient boosts the synthesis of important components at the epidermal junction which is where the hair anchors to the skin. This allows the actual hair follicle to stay more firmly attached to the scalp. In essence by stimulating cell communication and metabolism follicle anti-aging is promoted and anchoring molecules are rejuvenated. The final result being the stoppage of premature hair thinning and pattern baldness.

The chief ingredients of Procapil are tripeptide chains plus apigenin and oleanolic acid. Apigenin acts like a vasodilator enhancing blood flow in the scalp where oleanolic acid is a powerful antioxidant found to increase the hair's strength and longevity. The tripeptide chains are the centerpiece of this agent in that they help rebuilt the cellular network necessary for hair production.

- **More often than not these ingredients will be listed as Biotinyl GHK, Apigenin, and Oleanolic Acid instead of Procapil which encompasses all of the ingredients. Some manufacturers substitute various tripeptide chains and copper complexes.**

SOURCES FOR PROCAPIL

1. **MiN New York Topical Hair Loss Treatment, Shampoo, Conditioner, and Cleanser.**
   http://www.folica.com
   http://www.menessentials.com
   http://www.luxury4him.com
2. **Claude Bell Procapil**
   http://www.claudebell.co.uk
3. **Therapro**
   http://www.theraprohair.com
   http://www.sleekhair.com
4. **HairTec Tonic- Hair Fall Control Formula**
   http://www.2beaut.com
5. **Lakme K-Therapy Active Shampoo**
   http://store.hello-gorgeous.net
   http://www.fashionandbeautystore.com
   http://www.shampooline.com

PROGESTERONE

Progesterone is a hormone that when ingested orally does cause hair growth. The problem is that since it is a hormone, internal consumption in men can lead to female characteristics. Evidence though does exist that topically applied progesterone in hair products will reduce hair loss and promote hair regrowth. Used in this fashion systemic absorption is negligible. Since these products come and go in the marketplace, based upon demand, we are unable to suggest any in particular. Some products can be found at vitamin and nutrition stores or stores that cater specifically to hair care products. Progesterone taken orally is a prescription drug.

SOURCES FOR PROGESTERONE

1. **Found most often in large drug store vitamin sections.**
2. **Health and Nutrition Stores**
3. **Walmart Stores**
4. **GNC Stores**
5. **Various minoxidil and progesterone combination treatments.**
   http://www.jmsvitaminsonline.com
6. **Regenetresse Treatment For Women**

7. **CVS Drugstores**
8. **Walgreens**
9. **Shen Min Activator With Progestoplex**
   http://www.evitamins.com
10. **Natural Progesterone Cream**
   http://www.luckyvitamin.com
   http://www.soap.com
11. **Nugen HP – Expensive natural solution for women and men. Best price at:**
   http://www.onlyhairloss.com
   http://hairloss101.com
12. **Therapro Products**
   http://www.monsterhair.com
   http://www.alphabeauty.com
   http://www.theraprohair.com

PROPECIA-FINASTERIDE

Many people claim the "magic bullet" or pill for hair loss is the drug Proscar. Proscar is used in the treatment of prostate disorders, specifically benign prostatic hyplasia. Propecia (Finasteride) is the lower dosage tablet formulation of the same drug, which is marketed for baldness. Proscar the drug itself belongs to a group of medicines called enzyme inhibitors. In this case the enzyme inhibited being 5-alpha reductase. Excess amounts of this enzyme are directly linked to prostate enlargement. As pointed out earlier this particular culprit is also linked to male and female pattern baldness. Proscar and Propecia are both produced by Merck Pharmaceutical. These are prescription drugs.

The reason we recommend this particular drug is because it has been extensively tested. Evidence of side effects are few and those present tend to subside with extended usage. The lower dosage formula of the drug is even safer. The weaker dosage formula (Propecia) is dispensed in 1mg tablets used daily. Proscar on the other hand is prescribed in 5mg tablets. Effects of the drug do wear off with discontinuance.

If you have access to Proscar, users of the drug claim one 5mg tab taken weekly or quartering the pill and using it four times a week is sufficient to obtain results. Used in this fashion the drug becomes a highly affordable option. The 5mg pill is probably covered by medical insurance in some situations. Depending upon where purchased a yearly supply of Proscar can cost 100 to 150 dollars. Consultation with your doctor should take place to regulate your dosage and obtain the desired results.

- **The latest research out of Australia indicates that Proscar will produce excellent frontal hairline growth.**

- **Many hair restoration clinics now offer topical and oral treatments for hair loss. Proscar can be obtained in this manner if you prefer. Look in your local yellow pages.**

- **Since Propecia and Proscar both decrease hair loss everyday usage is not a requirement. Many people are quite happy just curbing their hair loss and use these products every two to three days. By doing so they maintain the hair they have, establish some regrowth, reduce their costs, and control any side effects that might appear.**

- **Benefits of Propecia may become apparent within three months. In double blind studies of 879 men experiencing hair loss eighty three percent had the same hair count or higher after two years, while using the 1mg. tablets. The average increase was one hundred and seven hairs based upon a measured one inch square in the vertex of the scalp. Other studies have reported significantly higher counts in the frontal areas.**

- **Oral dosage of 1mg. tablets of Propecia reduces serum concentrations of (DHT) dihydrotestosterone by sixty-five percent within a twenty-four period. This effect can last for up to four days in most users.**

- **This product is not prescribed or to be taken by women. Women of reproductive age are warned not to handle crushed or broken tablets of Propecia because of observed teratogenic effects in animals.**

- **Contrary to what most people think your local drugstores or discount chains tend to have the best prices for Propecia. If you let your doctor know you will be using a**

pill splitter he can write you a prescription for 5mg Proscar.

- **Merck's newest drug (Avodart) dutasteride has received approval for the treatment of benign prostatic hyplasia. Even though this medication is considerably more effective than Proscar for hair loss it has yet to receive approval as a hair loss treatment.**

- **Currently generic and brand Propecia plus Proscar can be found as cheaply if not cheaper in the United States.**

PRODUCT AVAILABILITY PROPECIA-FINASTERIDE

1. **Both Proscar and Propecia are available at your local pharmacies by prescription.**
2. **CanadaPharmacy.com**
   http://www.canadapharmacy.com
3. **Canada Drugs**
   http://www.canadadrugs.com
4. **North Drug Mart (Very Reputable)**
   http://www.northdrugmart.com
5. **Anagen Net**
   http://www.anagen.net/finasin.htm
6. **Canada Medicine Shop - Deals on 5mg Proscar**
   http://www.canadamedicineshop.com
7. **Deals For 1mg Finasteride**
   http://www.discountdrugsfromcanada.com
   http://www.canadadrugsonline.com
   http://www.globaldrugsdirect.com
   http://www.northwestpharmacy.com

PYGEUM

Pygeum is derived from the bark of an African tree of the same name. The actual extract has synergetic effects when combined with saw palmetto and nettles. For years, and still today, tribesmen of Africa have used this derivative in similar fashion to what the American Indians did with saw palmetto. Medical research has shown pygeum can reduce bloodstream DHT levels associated with benign prostatic hyperplasia. These DHT levels are related to hair loss. Effects are similar to such prescription drugs as Flomax and Proscar.

Pygeum's systemic effects upon the body are that it increases urine flow in those affected by prostate enlargement. Used in combination with nettles, inflammation of the prostate and excretory tract can be reduced. Herbal formulas often substitute pumpkin seed in place of pygeum. Pumpkin seed has a high concentration of naturally derived zinc and is cheaper but it lacks the anti-inflammatory qualities and DHT lowering capabilities of pygeum. Both though are extremely helpful to the prostate, just in a dissimilar fashion. One very big positive of pygeum and nettles is they are almost totally free of side effects.

As research has grown in the use natural alternatives for the treatment of hair loss the benefits of pygeum will likely become better publicized. Used together with saw palmetto these ingredients may prove to be one of nature's true gifts for hair regeneration.

- **One of the best sources for pygeum is Sundown Herbals Saw Palmetto Complex. This solution contains Pygeum, Zinc, Nettles, and Saw Palmetto in a very affordable combination. Similar European formulas can cost hundreds of dollars. Sundown's product can often be found at Walmart Stores. If you can't find this combination please look around for a suitable substitute.**

- **Prostate formulas containing Pygeum are always the best route. These combinations have widespread availability at most drugstores.**

SOURCES FOR PYGEUM

1. **Jarrow Formulas Ultra Saw Palmetto plus Pygeum**
   http://www.vitacost.com
2. **Enzymatic Therapy Products**
   http://www.swansonvitamins.com
3. **Solgar Saw Palmetto Pygeum Lycopene Complex**
   http://www.vitacart.com
   http://www.arnoldsupplements.com
4. **Solaray Pygeum & Saw Palmetto**
5. **Vitamin Shoppe**
6. **GNC Centers**

91

NATURAL HAIR LOSS INGREDIENTS GROUP Q

QUININE

Quinine is definitely not an ingredient to be ingested to combat your hair loss. On the other hand it does show significant results in retarding hair loss, thickening the hair you already have, reducing dandruff flaking, and stimulating some new hair regrowth. In this particular case though you're better off leaving the compounding to professionals. If you do make your own it is advisable to dilute by at least at twenty to one ratios with water.

To elaborate more on this toxic alkaloid it is derived from the Cinchona tree and has reported uses as early as the 17th century. Now it's chiefly classified as an antimalarial drug because it kills the organisms largely responsible for malaria.

SOURCES FOR QUININE

1.   **Klorane Quinine Shampoo**
      http://apothica.com
      http://skincarerx.com
      http://www.lovelyskin.com
      http://www.drugstore.com
2.   **Clubman Eau de Quinine Hair Tonic**
      http://www.clubmanonline.com

NATURAL HAIR LOSS INGREDIENTS GROUP R

RESVERATROL

Resveratrol is a polyphenol long associated with the life extending properties of grapes and blueberries. Isolated from these particular fruits it constitutes a potent inhibitor of the particular forms of DHT which are largely responsible for most hereditary hair loss. Grape seed extract also contains resveratrol along with other polyphenols.

Proponents of the usage of resveratrol have long maintained the beneficials effects can only be obtained through moderate wine consumption. The reality though is red grape skins contain the highest concentration of resveratrol.

- Resveratrol is again receiving renewed interest for its suggested life extending capabilities, which we were the first to publicize. It has also been reported these particular polyphenols if used regularly may be effective against type-two diabetes and help with weight loss. Amazingly some of the cheapest natural sources for this compound are red grapes, peanuts, peanut butter, boiled peanuts, and red grape juice if you can find it. Due to this recent up-tick in interest you can expect an increase in prices.

- Biotivia Resveratrol is often touted to be one of the best products in this category but it does carry an expensive price tag.

- With survey research many users claim they felt the most direct benefits from Resveratrol in comparison to all vitamins and herbs they had previously utilized.

SOURCES FOR RESVERATROL

1. The Vitamin Shoppe
   http://www.vitaminshoppe.com
2. VitaCost.com
   http://www.vitacost.com
3. Longevinex
   http://www.longevinex.com
4. Pure and Healthy
   http://www.pureandhealthy.com
5. Puritan's Pride
   http://www.puritan.com
6. ResVitale Resveratrol – GNC Stores

RETIN A

Retin A was introduced in 1969 as a topical solution for people doing battle with acne. It is a synthetic form of vitamin A. Subsequent research at the University of Pennsylvania showed that Retin A provided a host of skin renewing benefits.

Retin A works by stimulating the production of collagen between the skin's outer layer (epidermis) and inner layer (dermis). This additional collagen thereby reduces the wrinkling of the skin. Adding to this, Retin A encourages the growth of new blood vessels and accelerates the creation of new skin cells.

Formulations of this drug come in gel, liquid, or cream with varying degrees of strength. Newer combinations of the medication no longer result in dryness of the skin. In cases where dryness does appear, the skin adjusts in a short time frame.

What makes Retin A so interesting is that it works extremely well in tandem with other products. Scientists have known for years that combining this drug with minoxidil yielded astounding results. We advise consulting with a doctor to obtain your own prescription for this drug if you want to test out this true "hair growing" combination. The reason we point you in this direction is that most prepackaged formulations of minoxidil and Retin A that are currently available are somewhat expensive. Companies by virtue of being first to market these products will sell at a premium until competition emerges. An actual prescription of Retin A is very affordable and can last a considerable length of time.

Once you have consulted with your personal physician about what you would like to do we suggest making the combination yourself. This can be done by first applying 2% minoxidil and then following with the Retin A. As reports have confirmed the results might well astound you in nine to twelve months. Some people in a much shorter length of time. After that evidence indicates using this combo is only required six to eight months of the year, to maintain the desired results.

- **Retin A when combined with 2% minoxidil has proven effectiveness in reestablishing the frontal hairline. Based upon this fact combinations of the two should only be applied in the forward areas of the scalp. The reasoning behind this is that minoxidil alone is quite effective on the crown portions of the scalp.**

- **We do not recommend combining Retin A with higher strengths of minoxidil. Few reports on the safety of this combination have been investigated.**

- **Because of strict FDA parameters combinations of minoxidil with other ingredients will always be limited in** the United States. Such products would require new drug approval status in most cases. The exception is when dispensed by a doctor under Food and Drug Administration guidelines. These enhancements for minoxidil are marketed to increase the drug's effectiveness. Some are quite affordable and effective.

SOURCES FOR RETIN A

1. Doctor's prescription. Use with OTC 2% minoxidil. Should be used once daily at night.
2. Doctor Lewenberg's Formula
   http://www.baldspot.com
3. Remox and ProMox
   http://www.hairgrowthmd.com
4. Anagen Net
   http://www.anagen.net/prices.htm
5. Get Canadian Drugs
   http://www.getcanadiandrugs.com
6. MinSaw-A, International Antiaging Systems – Combination Retonic Acid, Minoxidil, Saw Palmetto Lotion. Should only be used at night.
   http://www.antiaging-systems.com
   http://www.aip-health.com
7. Spectral DNC
   http://hairloss101.com
8. Online Canada Rx
   http://www.onlinecanadarx.com
9. Shaltop-A Solution
   http://www.4cornerspharmacy.com
   http://www.unitedpharmacies.com

RETINOLS OF VITAMINS A AND D

These ingredients increase the cellular building capabilities of the skin and hair follicles. In simplified terms retinols are synthetic versions of vitamins A and D. They are listed as Retinyl Palmitate and Ergocalciferol on the packaging of products. Though not as potent as Retonic Acid they likewise are effective. Before purchasing a prescription for Retin A you first might experiment with over the counter products that contain these ingredients.

PRODUCTS CONTAINING RETINOLS OF VITAMINS A AND D

1. **Thicker Hair Thinning Hair Products**
2. **Biotene H-24 Thinning Hair Products**
3. **Amitee Hair Care Product**
4. **Nioxin Hair Loss Products**
5. **Retinol A Gel**
   http://www.jmsvitaminsonline.com
6. **Adama Clay Minerals Shampoo**
   http://www.vitasprings.com
7. **Dreamous Hair Renewal Shampoo and Conditioner**
   http://www.vitasprings.com
8. **Magick Botanicals Thinning Hair Shampoo and Conditioner**
   http://www.vitaminlife.com
   http://www.magickbotanicals.com
9. **Hairever Cleansing Scalp Treatment by Home Health**
   http://www.evitamins.com
   http://www.vitaminshoppe.com
   http://www.puritan.com

REVITA SHAMPOO

Revita shampoo is one of those products that really are so unique it deserves its own listing. Developed by DS laboratories it probably contains the greatest arsenal of DHT blockers, hair growth stimulants, vasodilators, anti-fungal, and scalp disorder agents that any one product can contain. Plus it improves the hair's fullness and vitality. Some of the listed ingredients are apple polyphenols, copper peptides, ketoconazole, spin traps, MSM, Rooibos, caffeine, amino acids, carnitine tartrate, Emu oil, and biotin.

SOURCES FOR REVITA SHAMPOO

1. **Revita Shampoo Store**
   http://revitashampoostore.com
2. **Salon Web**
   http://www.salonweb.com
3. **Hair Loss 101**
   http://hairloss101.com
4. **The Vitamin Shoppe**

http://www.vitaminshoppe.com

ROOIBOS

Rooibos is a member of the legume family and commonly means red bush. Grown only in a very small area of Africa its popularity is derived from the red tea processed from the plant. Chiefly known for its anti-inflammatory properties Rooibos is high in antioxidants. It is also the only known source for the polyphenol aspalathin. Rooibos is also the only tea that contains no caffeine and practically no allergic reactions have been reported with it.

In regard to hair loss Rooibos has been used for years as a hair loss preventative and hair growth agent. Even though this evidence has largely been anecdotal two recent studies involving over two hundred people concluded there was ample evidence to draw this conclusion. The studies concluded that anybody using Rooibos in a lotion of at least 5 ml. should see a significant reduction in hair loss and a measurable increase in hair growth.

- **We highly recommend any Rooibos shampoo as a natural treatment for hair loss. In many cases the products or ingredient is labeled Red Rooibos.**

SOURCES FOR ROOIBOS

1. **African Red Tea Rooibos Shampoo**
   http://www.africanredtea.com/rooibos-shampoo.html
   http://www.webvitamins.com
   http://www.supplementwarehouse.com
2. **Revita Shampoo**
   http://www.gnc.com
3. **Smart Organic Products**
   http://www.smartorganicproducts.com
4. **Segals Solutions**
   http://www.segalshairlosstreatment.com
5. **Herbal Glo See More Hair Deep Cleansing Shampoo, Conditioner, or Treatment**
   http://www.healthsuperstore.com
   http://www.herbalglo.com
   http://www.healthpalace.ca/brands/Herbal-Glo.html

NATURAL HAIR LOSS INGREDIENTS GROUP S

SAFFLOWER OIL

There are two versions of safflower each which produce different types of oil. One is high in polyunsaturated fatty acids (linoleic acid) and the other high in monounsaturated fatty acids (oleic acid). The predominant market being for the latter which is has lower saturates than olive oil. As we reported earlier these various essential acids are necessary for the healthy functioning of our bodies especially the skin and hair. The oil also contains high amounts of vitamin E and phytosterols. Its use has been documented since the days of the Egyptian dynasties.

In regard to hair loss the use of the oil is said to dilate the smaller capillaries within the scalp for enhanced blood flow. This in turn stimulates additional hair growth. Also since this oil has an abundant amount of the essential oils it acts as an excellent moisturizer for the scalp as claimed by many dry scalp sufferers. The oil can be utilized as a stand-a-lone product and applied to the scalp twenty minutes before shampooing.

SOURCES FOR SAFFLOWER OIL

1. **Klorane Safflower Oil Shampoo**
   http://www.adiscountbeauty.com
   http://www.stylebell.com
2. **Superbly Smoothing Argan Shampoo**
   http://www.kiehls.com

SALICYLIC ACID

You've probably heard very little about it but salicylic acid has been around for quite a while. Often used in the treatment of acne, psoriasis, and seborrhea its well-known for inducing a keratolytic effect upon the skin and scalp. This acid exhibits the same qualities as other salicycates, which is the ability to reduce inflammation and inhibit the immune response. Only recently though have scientists realized the capacity of this agent to retard the aging process.

Salicylic Acid by application to the skin and scalp is able to increase the renewal process of cells deep within the dermis. The advantage of this is that old cells are sloughed off at a quicker rate allowing cells to function at optimal levels. Basically in the area applied cells are rejuvenated.

In regard to balding use of salicylic acid can have multiple advantages for reducing hair fallout:

First, it increases the quality of the scalp's mantle by having the deepest pore cleansing capabilities of any OTC ingredient.

Second, its anti-inflammatory properties soothe the scalp thereby decreasing the immune response. This response which some scientists believe is linked to hair loss.

Third, by application the cells at the base of the follicle are regenerated at a quicker pace. This in turn re-energizes the small capillaries stimulating the growth of the hair shaft.

- **Shampoos containing this ingredient can substantially reduce hair loss if used at least twice a week. Combining with minoxidil after application can enhance hair growth results.**

- **Salicylic Acid is chiefly found in anti-dandruff shampoos and preparations.**

SOURCES FOR SALICYLIC ACID

1. **Neutrogena T/Sal Therapeutic Shampoo**
2. **Ionil Shampoo**
3. **Suave Dandruff Shampoo**
4. **Sebutone Shampoo**
5. **MG 217 Medicated Tar Free Shampoo**
6. **RegenePure DR Hair and Scalp Treatment**
   http://www.dermstore.com
   http://www.onlyhairloss.com

SARSAPARILLA

One method used by the American Indian to grow hair was by using the extract of the Sarsaparilla plant. Amazingly sarsaparilla contains an important male hormone necessary for hair growth called testosterone. Even though there is still some debate today as to whether this plant contains this male hormone, there is no doubt it contains one very similar to testosterone. If you have excess to this herb a hair wash composed of this root could prove very beneficial. Capsule versions of this herb are also available. Extracts isolated from the root are used to synthesize steroids such as progesterone. Sarsaparilla is found predominantly in the Western and Southwestern parts of the United States plus Mexico.

SOURCES FOR SARSAPARILLA

1. **Specialty vitamin and natural food stores.**
2. **Sarsaparilla Supplements
    http://www.iherb.com**
3. **The Vitamin Shoppe
    www.vitaminshoppe.com**
4. **Teo Tao Lemon Grass Shampoo and Conditioner**
5. **Himalaya Anti-Dandruff Shampoo
    http://www.himalayaherbals.com**
6. **Aubrey Organics Saponin A.C.C. Herbal Root
    Shampoo**
7. **Vitamin Life
    http://www.vitaminlife.com**
8. **Swanson Health Products
    http://www.swansonvitamins.com**

SAW PALMETTO

One product that is receiving a lot of press today is the herb saw palmetto. This saw tooth plant is native to the southeastern parts of the United States. For years herbalists have prescribed the berries of this plant for a variety of medicinal purposes. Chiefly amongst those being as a preventive and treatment for prostate troubles. Since saw palmetto affects the levels of testosterone its anti-androgen effects seem to lower DHT (dihydrotestosterone) levels in the body. This being the case many claims have arisen that saw palmetto halts hair loss and promotes hair growth. Unquestionably more study is called for, but undoubtedly many of these claims are true based upon anecdotal evidence.

Since this herb is known to have few side effects its popularity for the treatment of prostate troubles has grown enormously. Some physicians have gone as far as to say that the herb should be recommended by the FDA as a daily supplement for every man past the age of forty. Due to the substantial increase in prostate problems and cancer of this gland this advice might be well heeded. Bearing in mind that life expectancy of the average male continues to increase yearly, safe natural solutions such as saw palmetto should always be explored. The added benefits of halting hair loss, promoting regrowth on the scalp, increased stamina, and heightened libido could be viewed as "the icing on the cake," so to speak. Just remember if you want to test out this herb make absolutely sure you purchase the extract of the berries for potency. They can be readily purchased in pill form and extract is labeled on the packaging. Avoid buying formulas composed strictly of ground berries. They are ineffective against hair loss.

- **Monitor your results while using saw palmetto. We suggest employing a daily schedule upon initial consumption. After about six to eight weeks, reduction to a twice a week schedule or alternating days should be sufficient.**

- **The reason why saw palmetto works still perplexes medical authorities today. Research shows it neither shrinks the prostate nor reduces PSA levels, such as in the case of Proscar. In one large French study, which tested saw palmetto on over one thousand patients, symptom improvement was exactly the same as when using Proscar. In this study there were absolutely no reports of sexual impairment while using this herb.**

- **We highly suggest testing out saw palmetto before trying a prescription drug such as Proscar. This herb can be found rather cheaply if you look around enough. Results may be even better when combining with either Evening Primrose Oil or Borage Oil. More information on these two herbs can be found in our section related to essential fatty acids.**

- **One of the newest claims that have arisen about saw palmetto is that it may be much more effective in combating baldness than has previously been suspected. Empirical research now suggests that used once in the morning and once at night may produce hair growth in** about three months. Apparently this method allows reduction of DHT levels in serum cholesterol enough to trigger this regeneration. This phenomenon seems to rival the effects produced by more expensive prescription drugs. Since as stated earlier this herb can be purchased in quantity fairly cheaply and has few side effects, savings to the consumer can be significant. Some people do use 2% minoxidil in this regime for optimal results.

SOURCES FOR SAW PALMETTO

1. Prolamex
2. Sundown Herbals Saw Palmetto Complex
3. Walmart – Vitamin section.
4. CVS Drug Stores - Rated high for fatty acid and sterol content.
5. Regenepure NT
   http://www.regenepure.com
6. Tigi Bed Head Clean Up For Men Daily Shampoo
   http://www.sleekhair.com
   http://www.beautyofasite.com
7. Solgar Saw Palmetto - Rated high for fatty acid and sterol content.
8. Hair Stimulator Products
   http://shop.hlpcproducts.com
9. Nutra IQ Saw Palmetto Shampoo
   http://www.nutraiq.com
   http://www.hbees.com
10. Bianca Rosa Hair Loss Shampoo
    http://www.zooscape.com
11. Grow Shampoo
    http://www.growshampoo.com
12. Saw Palmetto Shampoo
    http://www.sawpalmettoproducts.com/sawpash.html
    http://www.vitamins-and-herbals.com
13. Min (DHT Blocking) Shampoo for Thinning Hair
    http://www.salonweb.com
14. Hair Fitness Shampoo
    http://www.healthandbodyfitness.com/
    http://www.webvitamins.com
15. Herbal Glo Advanced Thinning Hair Treatment – Saw Palmetto plus an excellent assortment of additional

ingredients.
http://www.healthsuperstore.com
16. **Boost Super Stimulating Shampoo and Conditioner**
http://www.worldofhair.com/hair/thinning.htm
17. **Pilexil Chute Shampoo**
http://www.shopmania.co.uk
18. **Corvinex Hair Nourishing Shampoo**
http://hairloss101.com
19. **Avalon Organics Biotin Shampoo**
http://www.vitacost.com
http://www.avalonorganics.com

SCALP ROLLERS

Scalp rollers are an invention that dates back hundreds of years. The theory behind all types of these rollers is to essentially stimulate the blood flow and micro-circulation within the scalp by massaging it with a roller type device. Many theorists believe that scalp massage methods are the only true way to stimulate hair growth and argue that increasing blood flow within the scalp is the purpose of about every hair loss product. Proponents of hair rollers also argue that these devices when used on a daily basis can lead to new capillary growth. This in turn enhances scalp circulation even more leading to better growth of the existent hair follicles. The newer devices utilize magnets, rows, and even needles to further enhance their effects and those of minoxidil. Marketers of these products also argue that these devices, unlike most hair loss products, only need to be purchased once unless you somehow loose it. That in turn could save you thousands of dollars. The added benefit of these devices is some people claim it returns the hair to its original color if you're suffering from gray hair.

- **These devices are particularly helpful where there is a traceable blood circulation problem as the result of thyroid conditions, medications, or chemotherapy. Some hair transplant surgeons also recommend these devices.**

- **Needle type rollers used in combination with minoxidil can be particularly effective when used in selected areas such as the frontal hairline.**

- **Needle rollers utilize some of the same principles as Retin A in that they stimulate collagen production.**

SOURCES FOR SCALP ROLLERS

1. **Microneedle Therapy System**
   http://www.microneedle.com/main/index.html
   http://www.ebskin.com
2. **Mag-Gro**
   http://www.rollyourscalp.com
   http://www.salonweb.com/mag-gro/
   http://www.onlyhairloss.com/mag-gro/
3. **Scientia Scalp Roller**
   http://www.derma-rollers.com
4. **Nanogen Scalp Roller**
   http://www.nanogenhair.com
   http://www.nanothick.com

SEA KELP

Kelp or seaweed is an extremely rich source of vitamins. To be accurate about all of the major nutrients plus minerals and amino acids. For years sea kelp has been used as a food source, preservative, flavoring, and additive to cosmetics and toiletries. Kelp contains in quantity most of the B-vitamins plus biotin, niacin, methionine, and inositil. All of the mentioned supplements being essential for hair growth. Since these vitamins are derived naturally it makes for an excellent ingredient for hair care products. Kelp is said to stimulate the on-off switch for hair growth in the follicle.

SOURCES FOR SEA KELP

1. **Pro Vitamin Hair Loss Treatment**
2. **Wildly Natural Seaweed Argan Shampoos and Conditioners**
   http://www.seaweedbathco.com
3. **John Allan's Ocean - Daily Nourishing Hair Shampoo**
   http://www.luxury4him.com
4. **Vitamin and Herbal sections of various stores.**
5. **La Source Volumizing Seaweed Shampoo**
   http://www.crabtree-evelyn.com
6. **Jack Black True Volume Thickening Shampoo with Expansion Technology, Basil, and White Lupine**
   http://www.getjackblack.com
   http://www.luxury4him.com

7. **Jason Natural Sea Kelp Shampoo and Conditioner**
   http://www.vitacost.com
   http://www.jasoncosmetics.com
8. **Rusk Deepshine Sea Kelp Shampoo and Conditioner**
   http://www.webbeautystore.com
9. **Bumble and Bumble Seaweed Shampoo and Conditioner**
   http://www.joybeauty.com
   http://www.bumbleandbumble.com
10. **Biolage Hydrating Shampoo and Conditioner**
    http://www.haircareusa.com

SEMODEX

One more exciting products to enter the marketplace was Semodex. This formulation being a development of Nioxin Hair Care, one of the most recognized names in hair loss research. Nioxin's extensive testing showed a linkage between certain mites found in follicles of balding individuals as opposed to scalp's experiencing no hair loss. These mites known scientifically as Demodex Follicularum generate lipases, which can directly affect hair reproduction. Pursuing these findings Nioxin developed products to eradicate and control these mites thereby decreasing these lipase growth inhibitors. Voila, we have Semodex, an over the counter offering with gratifying results.

Semodex incorporates a three-step program for fighting hair loss, which includes cleansers for eradicating the bacteria. Shampoos and conditioners are also included for maintenance of your results and further control of these lipase-producing culprits. And if you're wondering most over the counter hair care ingredients have little value in combating these mites.

Nioxin has a well-deserved reputation for creating quality products with high-grade ingredients and these should prove to be no exception. The ingredients are compatible with many hair types. Nioxin's approach may indeed become a breakthrough for dealing with baldness.

- **This product may has largely been discontinued with many dealers and replaced with Nioxin's system approach to hair loss. Many shampoos utilizing piroctane olamine now incorporate a similar approach.**

SOURCES FOR SEMODEX

1. **Nioxin's products are typically sold at leading men and women's hair salons. They are not usually found in retail outlets.**
2. **Skin-Beauty**
    http://www.skin-beauty.com/nioxin-kits.html
3. **Nutri-OX - Lower cost alternative to Semodex.**
    http://www.sallybeauty.com
    http://www.cachebeauty.com/hair_loss.htm

SHIKAKAI

Shikakai or Acacia Concinna is derived from a small shrub-like tree native to India. The name literally means "fruit for the hair". For years the pod like nuts of these trees has been utilized as a cleanser for the hair and scalp. Known for its astringent qualities it has been reported as an effective treatment for dandruff and hair loss.

The active ingredients in Shikakai are saponins, which are natural detergent like compounds. The advantage here is that these substances biologically attach to cholesterol so when water is applied cholesterol is naturally rinsed from the scalp.

SOURCES FOR SHIKAKAI

1. **Herbal Shikakai Shampoo**
    http://www.pureayurveda.com/haircare.html
2. **Shikai Shampoo**
    http://www.amerilifevitamin.com
    http://www.smallflower.com
    http://www.shikai.com
    http://www.drugstore.com

SILICA

One common mineral that is often overlooked as a hair loss preventative is the mineral silica. Popular in Indian Ayruvedic medicine and among naturopaths' usage seems to be limited to facial cosmetics, in most parts of the world. Among the previously mentioned dispensers of this compound there is a definitive description of a silica-lacking individual. Accordingly the "silica patient" is often a very chilly person, who tires quickly, suffers from acne, hair loss, and is a profuse sweater. Hence in theory silica taken internally can eliminate some of these indications. Male and female pattern baldness being one of these manifestations. Cosmetics containing silica serve as excellent exfolliants for removal of dead skin cells and debris on the body's surface.

The name silica is derived from the early Greeks who used it as an antidote for poisons. Appropriately their definition meant "To draw forth" which is exactly what silica seems to do. Amazingly when applied externally this mineral somehow gives the appearance that hair follicles are rejuvenated. Whether this is happening or not is open to a wide range of debate. Some popular "hair farming" techniques use these ingredients and swear by them. No empirical evidence is available to substantiate these claims one way or the other. The positive in this case is that most silica-enhanced merchandise is fairly cheap, so testing its benefits shouldn't be too costly.

- **Soviet scientists have reported that crushing silica tablets and mixing with your daily shampoo is an effective hair loss preventative.**

SOURCES FOR SILICA

1. **GNC Stores Natural Silica Products for the Hair and Skin**
2. **Sundown Vitamins Silica Supplements**
3. **Nature's Bounty Silica**
4. **Jason Thin-to-Thick Shampoo and Conditioner**
   http://www.supplementwarehouse.com
   http://www.jason-natural.com
5. **Image Shine Plus Silica Shampoo and Conditioner**
   http://www.sleekhair.com
   http://www.haircarechoices.com
6. **Boost Shampoo and Conditioner**
   http://www.worldofhair.com/hair/thinning.htm
7. **Barex Silicone Treatment Shampoo**
8. **Avanti Silicon Mix Shampoo**
   http://www.beautyofnewyork.com
9. **Prairie Naturals Harvest Moon Silica Shampoo**
   http://www.aviva.ca

SOD

Superoxide Dismutase (SOD) is an enzyme that repairs cells and reduces the damage done to them by superoxide, the most common free radical in the body. This ingredient is most often combined with an array of other growth stimulants in hair loss products. Studies have shown that SOD acts as both an antioxidant and anti-inflammatory in the body, neutralizing the free radicals that can lead to wrinkles and pre-cancerous cell changes. SOD levels in the body have been shown to decrease with aging. As noted hair loss researcher Dr. Peter Proctor has stated this decline in SOD levels is one of the primary factors in male and female pattern baldness. To elaborate more this excess DHT in the hair follicle causes specific immune and inflammatory responses that can be reduced with SOD. This in turns deters hair loss and stimulants growth of dormant follicles. It can be either ingested or applied topically to achieve its results. Products such as Folligen and Tricomin mimic copper SOD.

Superoxide Dismutase helps the body utilize zinc, copper, and manganese. There are two types of this enzyme, one being copper/zinc SOD and the other being manganese SOD. Each type of SOD plays a different role in keeping cells healthy. Copper Zinc SOD protects the cells' cytoplasm, and manganese SOD protects their mitochondria from free radical damage. SOD is found in barley grass, broccoli, Brussels sprouts, cabbage, wheatgrass, and most green plants. The body needs plenty of vitamin C and copper to make this natural antioxidant, so be sure to get enough of these substances in your diet as well.

SOURCES FOR SOD

1. **Supplement Spot SOD Cream**
   http://www.jmsvitaminsonline.com
2. **Corvinex Extra Strength Hair Growth Serum**
   http://www.corvinex.com
3. **NanoGaine Hair Growth Factor Treatment**
   http://www.nanothick.com
4. **Nano Shampoo**
   http://www.drproctor.com
   http://www.onlyhairloss.com
5. **Alterna Life Solutions Clarifying Shampoo**
   http://www.hairproducts4me.com
   http://www.skinstore.com

SOPHORA ROOT

One of the sleeper ingredients for treating your thinning hair are the extracts of the Sophora root. Long a staple of Chinese medicine three recent studies indicate the flavescens, within this herb, when applied topically are potent DHT inhibitors. Likewise these compounds are also capable of increasing the blood flow to the minute capillaries that supply the hair follicles. By performing both of the mentioned the anagen cycle (growth stage) of the hair is substantially increased. Scientists consider the elongation of this phase to be an absolute essential in delaying pattern baldness.

The extracts themselves are derived from the Sophora shrub which is native to Japan, China, Korea, and Russia. Similar too many of the Chinese herbs that combat hair loss, by improving the liver's functioning, this root also enhances this organs processes.

SOURCES FOR SOPHORA ROOT

1. **Seskavel Lotion**
    http://www.sesdermausa.com
2. **Hyssop Organic Brown Rice Moisture Shampoo**
    http://www.evecare.com

SORBIMACROGOL OLEATE AND SORBIMACROGOL STEARATE

Sorbimacrogol Oleate and Sorbimacrogol Stearate are high-grade surfactants derived directly from fatty acid esters. The only distinctions between the two being that in the stearate form the acids are saturated and in the oleate form they are unsaturated. Plus the oleate form having greater viscosity is better suited for compounding or dilution. The theory behind the use of these ingredients is that when applied to the scalp their absorption triggers both a histamine reaction in the skin and emulsifier action upon the scalp. This emulsifying action breaks up cholesterol formation necessary for the formation of the enzyme 5-alpha reductase. As explained earlier, this enzyme being a catalyst in causing hair loss. The histamine release, as also mentioned, is very similar to the irritation experienced after an insect bite. With the bite are the tingling, burning, and swelling caused by the histamine release, as blood is drawn to the affected area. This blood flow likewise is essential to the nourishment and growth of hair follicles upon the scalp.

In scientific terms three essential processes take place when these ingredients are applied to the scalp. These are all necessary for the growth of hair.

1. **Cholesterol and dihydrotestosterone are removed from the skin.**
2. **Release of histamine (growth factor) takes place.**
3. **Reversal of some of the prior genetic activities which bring about hair loss.**

Many people claim these compounds are an answer to baldness but as with many claims individual results can vary dramatically. As one university study showed the value of these products has probably been tremendously underestimated. It further stated that these ingredients could be an effectively cheap method for halting hair loss if not substantially prolonging or arresting the appearance of baldness indefinitely. The findings were based upon a regime of weekly usage. It was even noted in the study the mystery of why FDA approval has never been sought for these particular ingredients, as a hair loss preventive.

What's nice about these products is that they can be diluted, up to an eight to one ratio, without reducing their effectiveness. This allows the user to customize these ingredients to their own specifications. With the simple addition of water you can make your own shampoos and conditioners, tailored to your own specific needs. Many people have raved for years about the various horse mane and Helsinki products that employ these ingredients. What might shock you is how clean these products can actually make your hair and scalp feel upon using them.

- **These products are also referred to as the Polysorbates. Look for the ingredients Polysorbate 80 or 60 on the packaging before you purchase.**

- **When using products composed entirely of these two ingredients they should be applied directly to the scalp and allowed to sit for ten minutes or longer. Once this is done apply water and lather, similar to any shampoo. Then rinse.**

- **Suggested usage patterns for these products are twice a**

week.

- **Many companies offering these products commercially diminish their effectiveness with heavy dilution. We do not recommend exceeding the suggested eight to one ratio we have elaborated upon. This should ensure your results.**

PRODUCTS CONTAINING SORBIMACROGOL OLEATE AND SORBIMACROGOL STEARATE

1. **Polysorbate 80 Shampoo**
   http://minoxidildirect.com
2. **Polysorbate 80**
   http://www.recapturehair.com
   http://wholesalehairproducts.com
   http://www.lotioncrafter.com
   http://www.makingcosmetics.com
3. **Herbal Glo Thinning Hair Formula**
   http://www.hbees.com/herbalglo.html
   http://www.beautynaturally.com/hair.html
4. **Nioxin Hair Care Products**
5. **Rogaine Shampoos**
6. **Inner Shampoo**
   http://www.life-enhancement.com

SOY ISOFLAVONES

Soy isoflavones are one of the more popular ingredients in the diets of Asian populations but one of the most under-utilized nutrients in Western cultures today. Multiple studies have substantiated the fact that the incidence of pattern baldness increases in these Eastern cultures, once exposed to a Western diet lacking in these soy isoflavones. Add to this the evidence that the occurrence of cancer and heart disease also increases and you begin to realize just how potent these particular isoflavones are.

Soy to elaborate falls into a group of hormone-like compounds derived from plants known as phytoestrogens. The two predominant isoflavones in this phytoestrogen being genestein and diadzein. What's even more interesting is that this plant also contains known anti-cancer agents such as protease inhibitors, phytate, saponins, and phytosterols.

That's quite an accomplishment for one small plant.

Genistein in particular seems to compete with the body's own naturally occurring estrogens for absorption by the bodies' estrogen receptors. This is of particular significance to women because this competition seems to lower the incidence of breast cancer. Basically this particular soy isoflavone acts as an anti-estrogen preventing the more naturally occurring estrogens from reacting. Since the growth of breast cancer is estrogen dependent soy in effect may lower the incidence of this devastating cancer. As one study pointed out, women in Korea who regularly consume soy had close to twelve times less the occurrence of breast cancer than comparative female populations in the United States.

In regard to pattern baldness the consumption of soy seems to regulate bad cholesterol binding with enzymes in the scalp necessary for the production of DHT. By lowering overall cholesterol levels while at the same time decreasing LDL optimal conditions for hair growth are maintained.

- **This ingredient excites us probably more than most in its ability to combat hair loss and possibly slow the incidence of breast cancer in women. It's a natural food with numerous benefits.**

SOURCES FOR SOY ISOFLAVONES

1. **Soy Isoflavones can be found in capsule form in many stores today and will be labeled as such.**
2. **Soy Milk with Calcium - Particularly good for women with the addition of calcium, for prevention of osteoporosis.**
3. **Soy based products and flour. Check package labeling for assurance of actual soy.**
4. **Lamas Soy and Baobab Hydrating Shampoo and Conditioner**
   http://www.peterlamas.com
   http://www.soap.com
   http://www.drugstore.com
5. **Tofu**
6. **Fresh Soy Shampoo**
   http://www.fresh.com

7. **Origenere Shampoo for Thinning Hair**
   http://www.origenere.com
   http://www.hairenergizer.com
8. **Healthy Sexy Hair Soymilk Shampoo and Conditioner**
   http://www.sleekhair.com
   http://www.thebeautyplace.com
9. **Bellance Soy Protein Shampoo and Conditioner by Mill Creek**
   http://www.houseofnutrition.com

SOY MILK

Since you were young you mother always told you to drink your milk. The reason being is that milk fortifies the bones with its rich source of calcium. Now there's proof that by consuming soy milk you can reduce your hair loss.

Soy milk accomplishes its reduction in hair fallout through it's many complex isoflavanoes, in particular equol. Equol similar to Propecia reduces certain forms of DHT within our bodies that are largely responsible for hereditary baldness. The caveat here is even though soy products have shown an ability to combat hair loss plus an array of cancers it is still a nutritional approach for dealing with thinning hair. In effect you can't maintain an unhealthy lifestyle and expect to benefit solely from one form of supplementation.

SOURCES FOR SOY MILK

1. **Dairy sections of most food stores.**
2. **Peter Lamas Soy Hydrating Shampoo**
   http://www.peterlamas.com
3. **K&K Soy Products**
   http://kksoyproducts.com
4. **Healthy Sexy Hair Soy Milk Shampoo**
   http://store.hello-gorgeous.net

SPIRONOLACTONE TOPICAL

Spironolactone, often referred to by its brand name Aldactone, is a potent steroid drug that inhibits the action of aldosterone within the human body. When prescribed orally it causes the kidneys to excrete salt and fluids while retaining potassium. Medically it is known as a potassium sparing medication that promotes the output of urine (diuretic). The drug itself is utilized to counter-effect excessive salt and water retention within the kidneys which is often seen in heart failure and cirrhosis of the liver. To say the least it is a very potent oral medication that has increased the life expectancy of many, especially those unfortunate enough to be faced with cardiovascular disease. Spironolactone is undeniably one of the more researched drugs, for safety of purpose, because of the aforementioned conditions. It is indeed a miraculous drug in many respects.

Since numerous studies had been done regarding this drug it became obvious to researchers that it did possess anti-DHT properties that promoted hair growth and halted hair loss. The enigma being that anything as potent as Spironolactone should obviously never be used orally to treat hair loss. This is especially true since the medication itself is seldom used beyond short periods of time.

Topical Spironolactone came about because of the observed effects of the oral medication in patients. Researchers theorized that with the proper delivery system the medication could induce hair growth when applied to the scalp. Even though the verdict is still out on this version of Spironolactone, it has shown great promise in treating frontal hair loss.

- **Spironolactone should never be used orally to induce hair growth. The side effects could be potentially dangerous when used for a sustained period of time. Topical formulations have proven themselves to be far safer than minoxidil with regard to systemic absorption.**

- **The availability of topical Spironolactone is somewhat limited so you may have to search the Internet to find it. If you are able to obtain it you should look for odorless versions of the product.**

SOURCES FOR SPIRONOLACTONE TOPICAL

1. **Hair Loss Talk**
   http://www.hairlosstalk.com
   http://www.heralopecia.com
2. **Remox**
   http://www.anagen.net

3. **Wholesale Hair Products**
   http://www.wholesalehairproducts.com
4. **Topical Spironolactone**
   http://www.cemproducts.com
   http://www.medicalspecialists.co.uk
5. **Online Pharmacies via Internet**

SWERTIA CHIRATA EXTRACTS

Swertia Chirata is an interesting ingredient in that it has long been accepted as a hair growth agent and hair loss preventative but has never been solely utilized in any one product. It seems to works it best when combined with other hair loss compounds. The topical application of the extracts increases blood circulation in the scalp while sustaining the anagen phase of the hair growth cycle. It accomplishes this by irritating the areas at the bottom of the follicle into further production. Interestingly enough the extracts of this plant, which contain glycosides, are often used in Ayruvedic and Chinese medicine to treat diseases of the liver. It is a long held belief among practitioners of these oriental disciplines that all hair loss is related to the malfunctioning of the liver. The extracts also contain xanthones which are reportedly effective against malaria and tuberculosis. This herb also goes by the name Chirayata.

SOURCES FOR SWERTIA CHIRATA EXTRACTS

1. **Billy Jealousy Fuzzy Logic Hair Strengthening Shampoo**
   http://www.beauty.com
   http://www.cosmeticsnow.com
2. **John Allan's Thick Shampoo**
   http://www.themensparlor.com

NATURAL HAIR LOSS INGREDIENTS GROUP T

TAR SHAMPOOS

One group of ingredients that numerous people have found to be curiously effective in treating hair loss is products containing the various forms of tar. For years tar has been used as a cure-all for psoriasis, seborrhea, dermatitis, and eczema, plus the accompanying ills that surrounds these conditions. Since tar acts as an excellent cleanser, scales and flakes common to these conditions are eliminated from the scalp. This allows the follicle to reproduce under optimal conditions. Even though none of the previously mentioned afflictions has ever been fully linked to hair loss, treatment of these conditions often leads to an improved state of the hair and scalp. Similar to the sorbates, tar removes excess sebum and cholesterol that accumulates in and around the follicle. Since tar is processed in numerous ways there are quite a variety of products to choose from.

- **The amount of tar used in each of the following listed products varies by manufacturer and formulation. The actual percentages are listed on the packaging. In general the darker the color of the contents the greater the amount of tar used. The products also will list varying times to be left on the scalp. This is done to allow for the softening or loosening of the scales and flakes. Tar also generates a keratolytic (drying) effect that lessens sebum production.**

- **Some of the newest research indicates shampooing more frequently particularly with any dandruff shampoo does lessen hair loss.**

- **Tar products containing the chemical Dithranol can be the most effective DHT blockers for hair loss. But don't be concerned if you can't find it. Products containing this ingredient are few and far between.**

- **The suggested use pattern of these products is once or twice a week.**

PRODUCTS CONTAINING TAR

1. **Neutrogena Tar Shampoo**
2. **Pentrax Tar Shampoo**
3. **Herald Tar Shampoo**
4. **Denorex Shampoo**
5. **Tegrin Medicated Shampoo**
6. **DHS Shampoo**
7. **Hask Medicated Tar Shampoo**
8. **Pentrax Gold Shampoo**
9. **K-mart Tar Shampoo**

10. **MG 217 Tar Shampoo**
11. **Walmart Brands**
12. **Walgreens Drug Stores**

TEA TREE OIL

This unique herb's popularity seems to grow with each passing year. Found almost solely in Australia it is touted as a powerful anti-bacterial agent. For years it has often been referred to as "a medicine chest in a bottle". Some of the uses for the oil range from acne, sunburn, psoriasis, eczema, to fungus infections. Studies show it may be as effective as benzoyl peroxide and cortisone, in the treatment of skin disorders. Some research has indicated it is powerful antagonist to the bacteria of staph. Though not specifically linked to promoting hair growth the antiseptic properties of this oil can prove highly beneficial to the scalp. Tea Tree Oil can be found in many high-grade shampoos and conditioners.

SOURCES FOR TEA TREE OIL

1. **Vitamin and herb stores.**
2. **GNC Stores.**
3. **Nature's Select Tea Tree Oil**
4. **Jack Black True Volume Thickening Shampoo with Expansion Technology, Basil and White Lupine**
   http://www.getjackblack.com
   http://www.luxury4him.com
5. **Kiehl's Tea Tree Oil Shampoo**
   http://www.kiehls.com
6. **Tea Tree Therapy Shampoo and Conditioner**
   http://www.herbalremedies.com/teatree.html
7. **J.R. Liggett's Tea Tree and Hemp Oil Bar Shampoo**
   http://www.jrliggett.com/
8. **American Crew Tea Tree Shampoo**
   http://www.healthyhairplus.com
9. **Jason Naturals Tea Tree Oil Shampoo**
   http://www.iherb.com
   http://www.webvitamins.com
   http://www.nutritionexpress.com/jason
10. **Natures' Gate Tea Tree Calming Shampoo**
    http://www.natures-gate.com
11. **Desert Essence Tea Tree Shampoo**

http://www.iherb.com/store
12.   **Paul Mitchell Tea Tree Special Shampoo**
http://www.bodycare2000.com

TOCOTRIENOLS

Tocotrienols are part of the eight related compounds in Vitamin E. In particular they are credited with antioxidant and cholesterol lowering capabilities. Normally these particular compounds are not found in inexpensive versions of Vitamin E products. With some of the newer research that relates to this vitamin it has been shown that these Tocotrienols are capable of neutralizing the effects of HMG-CoA reductase. This enzyme is necessary for cholesterol formation. By inhibiting this enzyme LDL cholesterol levels are significantly decreased.

Since these compounds are so effective in reducing externally and internally produced cholesterol they are becoming the new "buzz ingredients" in combating hair loss. If you desire to use these constituents of Vitamin E you can either do so directly by supplementation or using various hair care formulations that utilize them.

- **Recent U.S. research has indicated that usage above 400 IU of Vitamin E daily has no beneficial effect. We suggest limiting your use of all vitamin E products to between 100-400 IU daily.**

- **In a recent study the usage of a patented Tocotrienols complex led to a 42 percent increase in hair regrowth in those suffering from male pattern baldness. This patented product, Carotech's Tocomin SupraBio complex has been reported to increase the oral absorption of Tocotrienols by 300 per cent.**

SOURCES FOR TOCOTRIENOLS

1.   **Health Food Stores**
2.   **Nioxin Herbal Supplement**
3.   **Nutriessential**
      http://www.nutriessential.com
4.   **Vitacost Tocomin SupraBio Palm Tocotrienol**

Complex
http://www.vitacost.com
5.   **Jarrow TocoSorb**
       http://www.vitacost.com
       http://www.swansonvitamins.com
6.   **Life Extension Super-Absorbable Tocotrienols**
       http://www.lef.org

TRIDAX PROCUMBENS

Tridax Procumbens is a plant that grows in India and is used in hair tonics in that country. Some preliminary American studies indicate topical and oral herbal treatments derived from this plant may indeed grow hair. Tridax has been widely recognized for years in Indian Ayruvedic medicine as a cure for baldness.

• **Ayruvedic practitioners typically recommend Bhringaraj (Brahmi Oil), Shikakai, Alma, and Ylang Ylang, to combat hair loss. These are not typical ingredients so the number of products to choose from is limited. Even though a number of non-US sites do sell these items we cannot recommend them because of potential security flaws in order forms.**

SOURCES FOR TRIDAX PROCUMBENS

1.   **Tridax Procumbens is not your typical herb so its availability is greatest at stores that specialize in the not so ordinary herbs and vitamins. Normally what you see on shelves will be Procumbens extract in capsule form.**

TURMERIC-CURCUMIN

One purely stand-alone treatment used in many parts of the world for hair loss in general and pattern baldness is Turmeric or Curcumin. There is no doubt that this ingredient reduces the mentioned but it usage tends to be confined to cultures where it is utilized as a condiment or in food preparations. Outside of that most people's exposure to it is chiefly through mustard where this ingredient gives it the distinctive yellow color. It has also achieved quite a following in the past few years as a natural treatment for psoriasis and arthritis. The only drawback seems to be for people suffering from gallbladder disease or gallstones where it should be avoided.

To give you a little background Turmeric it is a member of the Ginger family and finds heavy usage in curries and spicy dishes in the Middle East and Asian communities. It is used in many foods in the United States to add a distinctive yellow color. In medieval Europe it was called Indian saffron and used as a replacement for the much more expensive saffron spice. As one might expect India is the largest source of Turmeric with the cities of Erode and Sangli being the largest producers. Erode itself has long been referred to as Turmeric City or the Yellow City. The potential benefits of the active ingredient curcumin found in Turmeric are many and some are listed below.

a. Natural liver detoxifier.
b. May prevent metastases and a variety of cancers.
c. Natural relief for arthritis, psoriasis, and depression.
d. It is a known antiseptic and antibacterial agent.
e. Combining with cauliflower may prevent prostate cancer or the growth of prostate tumors.
f. It is a natural painkiller and cox-2 inhibitor.
g. May aid in weight management.
h. Helps with wound healing.

With regard to hair loss this ingredient draws many of its strengths from its anti-inflammatory properties. Plus when combined with resveratrol the two seemingly achieve a synergetic effect within the follicles that reduces TGF-b.

Many scientists as of lately now believe that this TGF-b factor may be the prime culprit in hereditary baldness. The caveat here is obtaining the purest turmeric to increase its absorption within the body thereby decreasing your present hair loss.

SOURCES FOR TUMERIC-CURCUMIN

1. **Life Extension Super Bio-Curcumin**
   http://www.vitaminshoppe.com
2. **Jarrow Formula**
   http://www.iherb.com
3. **Kal Turmeric and Resveratrol Combination**
   http://www.vitaminshoppe.com

4.   Aveda Invati System
http://www.aveda.com

NATURAL HAIR LOSS INGREDIENTS GROUP U-V

VANADIUM

Vanadium is another trace mineral usually found only in multiple vitamins. It is known to inhibit the formation of cholesterol in blood vessels. If you are looking for vitamins strictly formulated for the hair, check to see if this one is contained in the listed ingredients.

SOURCES FOR VANADIUM

1.   **Typically found in multiple vitamins. May be hard to find singularly.**
2.   **One Source Multivitamins - Walmart Stores - Very affordable.**
3.   **Centrum Multivitamins**

VITAMIN B-2 (RIBOFLAVIN)

Vitamin B-2 or Riboflavin has not been associated with hair loss until recently. Newer studies now indicate that this supplement used singularly may do more to reverse hair loss than previously suspected. Upon testing on small groups of men and women scientists found this vitamin alone could return hair loss to within normal ranges in most cases. This indeed was unusual because none of the participants in the studies showed any signs of a deficiency. The conclusion of the studies was that vitamin B-2 may have natural DHT inhibiting properties or it lowers the production of sebum.

To elaborate vitamin B-2 is one of the water-soluble vitamins that humans must obtain from nutritional sources or various OTC vitamin preparations. It is essential for cell growth and enzymatic reactions necessary to metabolize proteins, fats, and carbohydrates. By doing this the body is aided in antibody and red blood cell formation all necessary for healthy vision, skin, hair, and nails. A deficiency of this vitamin can exhibit itself in with itching, burning eyes, hair loss, cracks and sores in and around the mouth, bloodshot eyes, purplish tongues, dermatitis, retarded growth, digestive disturbances, trembling, and overly oily skin.

Vitamin B-2 can be found in brewer's yeast, almonds, wheat germ, polished rice, sunflower seeds, lamb's quarters, turnip greens, watercress, avocados, broccoli, collards, kale, dried apricots, mustard greens, spinach, most nuts, peas, dried dates, prunes, green beans, brown rice, raspberries, leaf lettuce, chard, lima beans, sweet potatoes, and soybeans.

Interestingly juicers often use many of the mentioned sources to retard hair loss. They maintain the vitamin is necessary for the boy's daily circadian rhythms and protection of gluthathione. In essence it promotes the healthy functioning of the liver.

SOURCES FOR VITAMIN B-2 (RIBOFLAVIN)

1. **Vitamin B-2 can be found just about anywhere but we suggest obtaining it by purchasing a B-Complex supplement.**
2. **Walmart Stores**
3. **Health and Nutritional Stores**
4. **GNC Stores**

VITAMIN B-6 (PYRIDOXINE)

Vitamin B-6 or pyridoxine is one of the busier vitamins in our bodies. Its chief function is helping the liver release glycogen whenever muscles need energy. It is also facilitates the conversion of linoleic acid to arachidonic acid (a more active fatty acid), in our bodies. This particular fatty acid keeps many of us from becoming obese. Additional functions of the vitamin are to aid in the synthesizing of nucleic acids, antibodies, and red blood cells.

The body does not store B-6 for lengthy periods of time like many of the other B vitamins. It is also one the few nutrients that many people are deficient in. The simple reason for this is because many people engage in constant dieting and subject themselves to considerable amounts of stress. B-6 is often destroyed in the processing of foods, pasteurization of milk, and by heat when cooking. So it's easy to understand why deficiencies are more common with this nutrient in comparison to others. One of its chief enemies among women is oral contraceptive pills.

Many newer studies do indicate this nutrient may be of greater value in combating hair loss and stimulating hair growth, than previously realized. Reasoning for this is not entirely clear but it may relate to the vitamin's ability to inhibit the histamine response in the scalp. It could also correlate with deficiencies that might have gone unrecognized for years. It's safe to say though if you're engaged in heavy mental demands, frequent exercising, or dieting you might not be getting enough of this vitamin and the result could be premature hair loss.

SOURCES FOR VITAMIN B-6 (PYRIDOXINE)

1. **Can be found just about anywhere vitamins are sold. Cheapest way to purchase is either singularly or in B-100 formulas. There are time release versions of this nutrient.**
2. **Centrum Vitamins**

NATURAL HAIR LOSS INGREDIENTS GROUP W-X-Y-Z

YUCCA

For years American Indians used yucca as a treatment for dandruff and hair loss. Plus if you're a student of history the American Indian, Aztecs, and Mayans all tried to combat these scalp conditions just as much as we today. To elaborate upon yucca it is native to the southwest and related to the Joshua tree. Various species of yucca are Spanish bayonet, soapweed, Adam's-needle, datil, whipple, and the dagger plant. Probably the most utilized portion of this botanical today is the root, which in reality is a mole. From this root are extracted powerful detergents known as saponins that can be made into natural soaps, body washes, and shampoos.

In relation to hair loss the extracts of the yucca root are reported to increase the growth rate and sheen of the hair by deep cleansing the scalp with these all-natural saponins. The key to why this plant may induce some hair growth on otherwise balding scalps may lay in the fact that the root is a very rich source of amino acids.

SOUCRES FOR YUCCA

1. **A Wild Soap Bar - Yucca Root Shampoo and Body Bar http://www.awildsoapbar.com**

http://www.greenlivingeveryday.com
2. Aubrey Organics Jojoba/Aloe/Yucca Shampoo
http://www.aubrey-organics.com
http://www.vitaminlife.com
3. Image Yucca Blossom Energizing Body & Shine Shampoo
http://www.brightonbeautysupply.com
http://www.goodlookingdiscounts.com
4. Yerba Hair Care
http://www.taosherb.com
5. Nick Chavez Yucca Root Shampooing Cream
http://www.beauty.com
6. Hobe Labs Energizer Treatment Shampoo
http://www.supplementwarehouse.com
http://www.swansonvitamins.com

ZINC FORMULA FOR HAIR LOSS

As research regarding zinc has increased various homemade topical formulations attesting to its effectiveness have begun to appear. Popularly referred to as Zix because of a combination of zinc sulfate and vitamin B-6, these formulas seem to have an increasing body of anecdotal evidence pointing to hair regrowth. An initial study with a limited number of participants did show very promising results with topically applied zinc, B-6 solutions. Unquestionably zinc is essential to hair growth and is an effective DHT antagonist. Various formulations applied to the scalp may indeed prove to be just the answer for hair loss. One such formula is listed below.

ZINC FORMULA SUPPLIES NEEDED

1. Four ounce bottle or two empty minoxidil bottles with eyedropper cap.
2. 5 - 50 mg. capsules of zinc sulfate
3. 6 - 20 mg tablets of vitamin B-6
4. 4 ounces of distilled water.* We suggest substituting 4 ounces of Folicure Leave In Conditioner, which is a liquid conditioner meant to be left on the scalp. It contains various beneficial ingredients for scalp penetration plus preservatives.

Once you've assembled the ingredients, crush the zinc

and B-6 capsules to a fine powder and combine with the distilled water or Folicure Conditioner. Now allow the ingredients to dissolve, which can take about three days. To use just shake thoroughly to further disperse the ingredients. Then apply as desired. The formula should be applied twice daily to the affected areas.

HAIR LOSS AND GROWTH SUPPLEMENTS

INOSITIL, CHOLINE, PABA, CYSTEINE, SELENIUM, AND ZINC

All of the above bold-faced vitamins are widely regarded, as must have vitamins for hair growth. The additional benefits of these vitamins in regard to other bodily functions would probably be to numerous to list, as more scientific evidence becomes available daily. The first three vitamins listed all belong to the B-vitamin group. The next Cysteine is one of the building blocks of hair formation and cell membrane stabilization. Plus with the last mentioned, selenium and zinc are trace minerals, which can halt free radical damage in the human body.

To elaborate more on each vitamin we'll first start with Inositil and Choline. These two vitamins can be found in their highest concentration in the brain area. Associated with making energy available to the body, studies have shown that a lack of these two nutrients can cause hair loss. In experiments using at least 1000 mg. of these vitamins hair loss was substantially retarded. Hair growth was also observed but not in all cases. Reports of graying hair darkening were documented, but likewise not in every case. Since both vitamins are fairly inexpensive when purchased at discount stores, they seem to be a bargain for curbing hair loss. Don't be surprised either if you notice an improvement in your memory. These nutrients have been associated with increasing recall of past events.

Following the above mentioned nutrients is another one of the B-vitamins commonly known as PABA (para-aminobenzoic acid). PABA primarily increases the body's resistance to the elements and reduces free radical damage in the body. Free radicals are widely recognized as the chief culprits in the aging process. PABA similar to Inositil and Choline has about the same results when it comes to hair loss. It is able to decrease the thinning process when used, produces some hair growth, and does darken some hair. As many of us well know, when

PABA is applied by way of suntan products, it protects the skin and hair against ultraviolet rays from the sun.

The next nutrient in our list is Cysteine. Hair is composed of about ten percent Cysteine. Use of this amino acid will increase the growth rate of your hair. So if you want to double your hair's growth rate this is the nutrient. Just remember if you're planning to use large quantities of Cysteine make sure that you use vitamin C with it.

The final two vitamins in this group are zinc and selenium. Both of these nutrients are widely found in anti-dandruff compounds available at retail stores. They are listed as zinc pyrithione and selenium sulfide on the packaging of the product. The purpose of the ingredients is to eliminate the free radical damage caused by the oxidation of fats on the scalp and in the body. By doing this the scaling, flaking, and itching associated with dandruff are reduced. Studies have shown that by utilizing these ingredients, in a weekly regime, hair loss can be substantially curtailed. This is by virtue of the cholesterol removing properties of these ingredients. Currently zinc is also receiving increased exposure because of its ability to halt the common cold or shorten its duration. Selenium on the other hand has been linked to a reduction in various forms of cancer.

- **Claims have arisen that zinc in topical and tablet form has greater value than previously realized in preventing hair loss. Indications are also that it may act in a short duration of time. Since zinc can often be purchased at less than two dollars for one hundred tablets its well worth experimenting with, if just purely for the purpose of reducing the amount of cold viruses you may catch. We suggest though limiting the dose to 10 mg, depending upon one's tolerance. Larger doses can lead to diarrhea and anemia. Zinc in the topical formulation is labeled zinc oxide.**

- **The B-Vitamins have been traditionally linked to curbing hair loss and promoting hair regrowth. Various proprietary formulas are available such as those made by Solgar, which are backed by extensive research. Many people use B-100 formulas or enhanced multiple vitamins for the same purpose. Avoid excessive amounts of vitamins A, D, and Iron in these formulas unless you** have a known deficiency. Iodine is also an absolute necessity for hair growth but deficiencies are rare, since this mineral is often found in ordinary table salt. Also using dry tablet formulations of these nutrients is preferable. Gel formulas may contain excessive amounts of estrogens.

SOURCES FOR INOSITIL, CHOLINE, CYSTEINE, PABA, SELENIUM, AND ZINC

1. Various OTC vitamins, supplements, and hair care products at local stores.
2. Head and Shoulders Shampoo
3. Selsun Blue Shampoo
4. Redken Intra Force System 1&2
   http://www.usabeautysupplies.com
   http://www.sleekhair.com
5. ZincPlex Scalp Care
   http://www.scalp-health.com
6. Nexus Danderrest Shampoo
7. Biotene H-24 Shampoo and Conditioner
   http://www.evitamins.com
   http://www.gnc.com
8. Nexus Biotin Cream
9. CVS Stores Zinc Oxide Ointment
10. GNC (General Nutrition Stores) Ultra Nourishair Vitamins
11. Sundown Vitamins for the Hair
12. Nexus Cysteine Shampoo and Conditioner
13. Hairtopia
    http://mp.hairboutique.com/
14. Hair Formula 37
    http://www.hairformula37.com
15. Therapro Mediceuticals – Good DHT blockers but pricey product line-up.
    http://www.evabeauty.com
    http://www.theraprohair.com
16. Home Made Zinc Formula
    http://www.advinfoprod.com/hair_loss_treatment_1.htm
    http://www.qdbd.com/hair_loss_treatment_1.htm
17. Kal Hair Force and Hair Kare

http://www.vitaminshoppe.com
18. **Solaray Hair Nutrients**
http://www.evitamins.com
19. **Head Start Supplements For Your Hair – May still be available at CVS Drug Stores.**
http://www.headstartvitamins.com

BOTANICAL AND HERBAL REMEDIES

APPLE CIDER VINEGAR, ONIONS, ROSEMARY, SAGE, NETTLE, HORSETAIL, AND CHAMOMILE

One of the cheapest methods for lessening hair loss, handed down through the years, is using apple cider vinegar. Similar to some of the other products mentioned apple cider vinegar reduces cholesterol formation on the scalp and sebum buildup with its deep cleansing properties. Upon application the scalp's acidity is reduced.

To use as a rinse add one tablespoon of apple cider vinegar to a quart of warm water and apply to the degree you like, which comes with experimentation. Used once or twice a week it will probably surprise you. Besides having cleaner looking hair you'll notice less dandruff and hair fallout with time. You will find that a tablespoon or less of the vinegar is quite sufficient.

This solution through the years has also been combined with various herbal ingredients such as rosemary, sage, nettle, horsetail, and chamomile to increase its potency. The suggested method is to steep the herbs in warm water, let cool, and apply as desired. A variety of hair loss shampoo now contain the mentioned ingredients so purchasing via that method is likely the most cost effective route.

Another technique used since the days of the early Egyptians to combat baldness is the use of onions. And to be specific any type of onion can be used, especially yellow onions. Onions are excellent for reducing cholesterol both internally and externally. Besides inhibiting sinus trouble, onions are an especially high source of Inositil and Choline, in their purest form. The significance here is being that these two vitamins are essential for hair growth.

To use. Squeeze the contents of some average size onions into a container or liquefy them with a blender. Now add about a tablespoon of apple cider vinegar to reduce the odors. Once done, cover the container and refrigerate overnight. This solution can be used immediately, if you desire to do so. When using this solution you should apply for ten minutes or longer and then follow with shampooing. Used once or twice a week you might be amazed at the results and how clean your scalp will feel.

- **The marketing catch phrases for these products are typically all natural ingredients or botanicals.**

- **Our advice is to look for shampoos and conditioners that contain the suggested herbs in retail outlets. The supply is numerous. If one does have a source for natural extracts of the recommended herbs, by all means try them.**

PRODUCTS CONTAINING VARIOUS NATURAL INGREDIENTS AND BOTANICALS

1. **Thicker Fuller Hair Products**
2. **Five Element Apple Cider Vinegar Fire Shampoo**
   http://morroccomethod.com
3. **Frederic Fekkai Apple Cider Vinegar Clarifying Shampoo**
   http://www.drugstore.com
   http://www.lovelyskin.com
4. **Matrix Systeme Biolage Hair Care Products**
5. **Nexus Diamtress Shampoo**
6. **Redken Hair Care Products**
7. **Mountain Ocean Hair Maximum Shampoo**
   http://www.swansonvitamins.com
   http://www.iherb.com
8. **Various Botanical Shampoos and Supplements**
   http://www.vitaminshoppe.com
9. **Aubrey Organics**
   http://www.aubrey-organics.com
10. **J.R. Liggett's Damaged Hair Formula**
    http://www.jrliggett.com/
11. **American Crew Thickening Shampoo**
    http://www.americancrewshop.com
12. **Lavaggio Prima Rosemary Leaf Shampoo and Treatment**

http://www.myworldhut.com
13. **African Formula Supergrow Moisturizing Cream Rinse**
http://www.pennherb.com/
14. **Wise Ways Herbals Apple Cider Rinses and Root Tonic**
http://www.luckyvitamin.com
15. **Lavaggio Prima Rosemary Shampoo**
http://www.ediblenature.com
16. **Just Natural Vinegar Rinse Cleanser**
http://www.justnaturalskincare.com
17. **ACV Apple Cider Vinegar Shampoo**
http://www.iwantthathair.com
18. **Bioforce USA Onion Hair Lotion**
theherbalhealthstore.com
http://store.theherbalhealthstore.com
http://www.herbspro.com

EASTERN THERAPIES

Since the early days of the Han and Ming dynasties Chinese herbs have been used for a variety of medical conditions. Passed down through the years by trial and error, many are still used extensively today. In Chinese folklore, herbs can return the body to its natural state of being. In the case of baldness these herbalists maintain that by allowing the kidneys and liver to function properly, hair loss can be prevented and graying hair can be darkened once again. Interestingly enough it is the liver's failure to neutralize excess testosterone in the blood stream that leads to elevated amounts of DHT in the scalp. As modern science has shown many of these herbs have powerful anti-oxidant capabilities. By preventing free radical damage to cells, various bodily functions can be enhanced for optimal performance. To fully understand why these herbs work makes for exceedingly interesting reading.

Listed below are some of the better known Chinese herbs used to treat baldness and graying hair. These are certainly not the only ones because herbalists choose from a wide list when prescribing treatments for hair loss.

GREEN TEA EXTRACTS "LIQUID JADE"

Green tea first became noticed by nutritionists and scientists as an explanation for lower death rates from cancer and heart disease in Asian cultures. Part of the reasoning was linked to green tea. Subsequent studies at the University of Minnesota involving 35,000 subjects did indicate that all teas, especially green tea extracts, protect against the initiation and promotion stages of cancer. Method of ingestion was predominantly in beverage form.

Green tea is high in polyphenols as exhibited by the green leaves. Polyphenols are naturally occurring substances found in plants that are best known for their role as antioxidants. Tests have shown that green tea and its polyphenols may be the most potent antioxidant that nature has revealed to us. Plus green tea extracts are even more powerful when taken with such supplements as vitamin E and zinc. Since these polyphenols do reduce bad cholesterol and DHT in the body, many people claim that ingesting green tea or taking the pill extracts will curb hair loss and facilitate hair regrowth.

Other research indicates green tea...
Guards against toxins from salmonella.
Fights the bacteria from dental plaque.
Protects the gastrointestinal tract plus its beneficial bacteria.
Has anti-ulcer properties.
Encourages anti-viral activity.

- **All tea contains polyphenols and may inhibit hair loss. Green Tea though has a much higher content of green polyphenols.**

GOTO KOLA

Among Taoists this is a reputed hair growth herb and brain tonic that increases longevity. It is said to open the "Crown Chakra" at the top of the head. To the Chinese this meant stimulating the blood flow in this area to increase the release of energy to the body and mind. Some research does validate this occurrence. Tightening of the skin in the scalp, as Taoists have suggested, may indeed decrease blood flow to small capillaries necessary for hair growth. Even though one can induce quick blood flow by cutting the scalp, it is the minute vessels that stimulate the hair follicles to grow. And this tightening of the skin layer above the skull may well be the reason for baldness in the crown and forehead.

HO SHOU WU

This herb is linked with slowing hair loss and darkening graying hair. The herb was named after the Chinese king (Ho) whose head (Shou) of white hair turned black (Wu) and regrew after using it. Hence the name Ho Shou Wu. The Chinese have always linked this herb with mysterious properties of rejuvenation. In the United States this herb is often referred to as Fo-Ti. Extracts of the plant do possess anti-bacterial qualities. This herb is used in modern China as a medical treatment for high cholesterol.

- **Chinese practitioners have long maintained the ability of Ho Shou Wu (Fo-Ti) to darken graying hair. Used three times daily results should become apparent in two months and continue to increase past this point. At worse you will likely see improvements in hair reproduction and cholesterol levels.**

HAN LIEN TSAO

Han Lien Tsao is traditionally known as the "ink vegetable", for its ability to darken hair. Taken internally or administering the extract topically to the scalp is said to promote hair growth. The primary ingredient of this herb amazingly is nicotine combined with large amounts of vitamin C and niacin. Nicotine used in this manner has been shown to reduce cholesterol on the scalp and in the body.

GINGKO BILOBA

For over 5000 years Chinese herbalists have prescribed the extracts of this tree for respiratory and circulatory complaints. Gingko derived from the tree of similar name is composed of two active components. These are glycosides and terpene lactones. Glycosides are powerful antioxidants, which inhibit blood clot formation in the body that could result in strokes and arteriosclerosis. The terpenes on the other hand primarily increase circulation to the brain and scalp areas. This positive increase in blood circulation extends even to the minutest capillaries supplying the hair follicles. When the hair root is well supplied with blood it is less susceptible to the miniaturization effect exerted on the follicle by DHT. Chinese herbalists maintain as long as the scalp is well supplied with blood it is very difficult for an individual to experience baldness. These terpines also increase the elasticity of the blood vessels enabling circulation to become more efficient. Recent research indicates that this herb may also enable nerve cell regeneration. Gingko Biloba is utilized in many Chinese hair growth formulas.

SOURCES FOR CHINESE HERBS

1. **Holistic Chinese Herbs**
    http://www.holisticchineseherbs.com
2. **Reminex for Gray Hair**
    http://www.reminex.com
3. **Kal Hair Force**
    http://www.evitamins.com
4. **Solaray Hairx – Shen Min alternative**
    http://www.a1supplements.com
    http://www.affordablesolaray.com
5. **GNC Stores**
6. **Bell Natural Superior Hair**
    http://www.evitamins.com
7. **The Vitamin Shoppe**
    http://www.vitaminshoppe.com
8. **Peter Lamas Chinese Herb Stimulating Shampoo**
    http://www.peterlamas.com
9. **Puritan's Pride**
    http://www.puritansale.com
10. **Salern Biokera Specific Falling Hair (Ginkgo Biloba Extract)**
    http://www.justbeautyproducts.com
11. **Deity of Hair Plant Shampoo for Hair Loss**
    http://www.justbeautysupplies.com
12. **Nu Hair - Hair Regrowth For Men/Women**
    http://www.luckyvitamin.com

OXYGEN UTILIZATION TREATMENT - JOGGING AND WALKING

One of the simplest if not cheaper ways to lessen hair loss is by engaging in a simple exercise program which increases the body's utilization of oxygen. Two Canadian and one British study have confirmed this. Volunteers in these investigations were asked to participate in simple exercise programs consisting of jogging and walking to test this hypothesis. Hair fallout rates were checked for a period of time before the participants were asked to begin these prescribed programs. Amazingly most of the participants showed a marked reduction in hair loss rates, with the vast majority showing a return to fully normal levels of hair loss. Indications were that a fifty-percent reduction could be expected in six to eight weeks. Even though this study showed no cure for baldness it did reveal the possibilities of retarding hair loss for many years.

The hypothesis of these studies was that increased use of oxygen could inhibit the hair loss process. It must be noted though, that many variables were not examined that could have influenced the results. This was pointed out in the final data. Undoubtedly decreased cholesterol levels, reduction in levels of stress, and increased cardiovascular fitness could be reflective factors of the actual exercise and vary causatively with each individual. But the increase in oxygen usage would have occurred with each person. The results albeit were clear, exercise apparently reduces hair loss in most individuals. Plus this increase in physical activity on a regular basis could delay the onset of "shiny dome" for quite a few years.

SUGGESTED EXERCISE PROGRAM FOR WALKING AND JOGGING

(Five Days a Week)
First Week
Walk one mile a day and jog a quarter of a mile.

Second Week
Walk a mile and a half a day and jog a half-mile.

Third Week
Walk two miles a day and jog three quarters of a mile.

Fourth Week and Beyond
Walk two miles a day and jog a mile.

- **All exercise programs should be entered with caution if you have known health problems such as diabetes, obesity, heart disease, liver, kidney, or muscular skeletal** problems.

- Don't let your ego or others push you beyond your capabilities to quickly. These are merely suggested programs. Always proceed at the rate you are most comfortable with. Remember professional athletes must work at programs many years just to achieve two minutes or two hours of optimal performance. Their physical prowess and muscles didn't develop overnight. The typical individual's profession is not fitness. Athletes are often surrounded by a wealth of trained health practitioners to keep them injury free. Anybody embarking on an exercise regime is bound to feel the aches and pains when starting out. Just don't overdue it.

- Preferably run or walk with a friend or partner in well-lit areas. This is important for safety and emergency reasons.

CALCULATIONS FOR JOGGING AND WALKING

- A typical school track will be a quarter of a mile in length.

- Most people walk a mile in twenty to twenty-five minutes.

- The typical individual jogs a mile in eight to ten minutes. Unless you've been training for at least two years very few people jog a mile in less than six or seven minutes unbelievable as this may sound. So if you're starting out and venturing across various terrains the best measurement is two and a half minutes of jogging is equivalent to a quarter of a mile. Where ten minutes of jogging equals about a mile. You can observe these times with a regular wristwatch or stopwatch.

- A rough estimate of the distance to be covered can also be calculated by tracing a route with the odometer in your automobile. This calculation is based on if you're planning to walk or jog on sidewalks and the course to be negotiated is near roads.

FEMALE SPECIFIC THERAPIES

Thinning hair, hair loss, and baldness are not maladies strictly confined to the male gender. Females are also susceptible to exactly the same culprits. The medical community and manufacturers of health and beauty aids have ignored this all too often. The irony of the situation is that excess DHT linked to baldness in men can be found in a like manner in women. This fact combined with hormonal changes that take place as women age, along with entering the childbirth years, can further intensify the loss of hair. Just as men find their hair to be their "crowning glory" women do also. Besides the fact that fewer women are actually bald compounds the stress of hair loss even more in females. Luckily the same ingredients that are helpful to men can be equally useful to women.

Since women are uniquely different from men it is always wise to consult with a physician or dermatologist first to determine if any medications or bodily changes might be creating the problem. With women the trouble could certainly have more of a biological basis than a genetically acquired one. Once this has been done a proper course of action can be determined.

Being repetitious about all of the amazing ingredients we have mentioned throughout these writings are just as suitable for women as men. Most of these mentioned products have been formulated so that they are not gender specific to any group. We particularly applaud such companies as Upjohn, Folicure, Nioxin, Nexxus, Herbal Glo, Redken, Jannsen, and Thicker Hair, who have products and pharmaceuticals appropriate for both sexes.

In regard to vitamins, minerals, and nutrients we recommend all women utilize a good multiple vitamin, B-vitamins, calcium, and particularly vitamin B-6. B-vitamin deficiencies are often more prevalent in females than once was realized. Plus calcium not only prevents future and present bone loss, it is also one of the essential building blocks of hair growth.

It is also important to point out that women often employ a wider range of treatments that can culminate in premature breakage of the hair follicle and weakening of the cuticle, if utilized to frequently. Hair coloring, permanents, and frosting do not per sec cause hair loss but they do tend to brittlize the hair shaft with time. Because the follicle is not basically porous the bonding of ingredients employed by these treatments can only take place by penetration of the cuticle. Another words the shaft is made porous to absorb the ingredients and achieve the desired results. Overuse though can create so much porosity the cuticle will split and then eventually break off. Normally this is not a problem with short hair because of the greater cutting frequency which scissors out the damage. In longer hair the resultant use of silicones to regulate the problem can cause a noticeable greasy build-up with time. So it is advisable to follow the suggested routines for touch-ups and full applications.

Another area to consider which places a considerable strain on the follicle is hair straightening. This process is innately harsher on the cuticle and scalp because of the chemicals involved. Overdone or used to often these substances can lead to severe hair breakage and temporarily halt hair reproduction. Generally you can spot this if you show thinning in the crown areas of the scalp. This doesn't mean this is the only area affected but the area where hair loss first becomes most visible. Longer hair on the sides of the scalps can mask the less obvious.

We also caution all women who may be pregnant as to the use of any agent for hair loss. It could have injurious effects upon the fetus in some cases. So an ounce of prevention is worth a pound of cure. It is worth noting that during pregnancy many women will experience hair loss. This should not be cause for alarm because it dissipates after childbirth. So don't let this become a source of your anxiety because having children can be stressful in and of itself. Hormone replacement is also available for women experiencing hair loss as a result of aging.

CALCIUM CITRATE, VITAMIN D, AND IRON

Since you were a young child you've been taught that calcium builds strong bones and teeth. Well guess what, it's also essential for the health of your hair. Even though this mineral can be found quite easily in various food groups and milk, the alarming rise in the incidence of osteoporosis shows many women are not receiving their daily quota of it. If you don't get enough calcium from the foods you eat your body automatically takes it from the bones. Too much of that happening and the result is thinning of the bones or sometimes bone spurs. One of the early signs in women that they may not be supplementing the body with enough calcium is hair loss on the scalp. This phenomenon seems to occur in many women in the early forties but can occur at any age. Calcium is also shuttled from the bones to maintain the nervous system, blood pressure, and heart rhythms. It's also necessary for the absorption of vitamin B-12.

What's interesting about calcium is that no matter how much you obtain of it in your diet you must have an adequate amount of vitamin D for it to be absorbed in your gastrointestinal tract. So if you're not spending an adequate amount of time in the sunlight make sure vitamin D is combined with the calcium to assure assimilation. If you are already using a multi-vitamin with vitamin D in it, then purchasing a formula strictly composed of calcium is the most cost-effective route.

How much calcium should you use? It varies with your age and how much you already obtain in your diet. Adequate amounts of this mineral can be found in regular, low-fat, and skim milk if you consume this beverage on a daily basis. If not calcium can be found in all dairy products, green leafy vegetables, broccoli, cauliflower, Brussels sprouts, and all dried peas and beans. The suggested consumption should be at least 1000 mg. a day if you're under 50 years of age and 1200 mg. if you're above 50.

What's the best form of calcium to use? Actually it's all good for you but studies tend to indicate calcium citrate is the most absorbable in your digestive tract. Most of the other forms of the mineral require digestive acids for absorption, where calcium citrate does not.

Iron is another mineral that plays a vital role in hair growth but like calcium it tends to only show up as a deficiency in women. When a woman loses iron as a result of trauma, poor diet, or heavy menstruation several things can occur. Among them, her body literally stops producing hair until she gets more iron. This phenomenon can even occur with regular menstruation and moderate anemia.

To compensate women can increase their daily intake of iron, which should be at least 18 mg a day. To facilitate the absorption of iron one should also use vitamin C.

- **Large doses of iron can darken the stools temporarily. Unless you have a known deficiency of iron, or a doctor has suggested otherwise, it is wise to keep the dosage below 30mg. In dosages above this sensitivities may produce digestive tract complaints in some.**

SOURCES FOR CALCIUM CITRATE, VITAMIN D, AND IRON

1. **Caltrate Calcium Citrate**
2. **Caltrate Calcium Citrate with Vitamin D**
3. **Sundown Vitamins Calcium Supplement**
4. **Iron Supplements can be found in many stores.**
5. **All milk and yogurt products.**
6. **Brick cheese, kelp, dark green vegetables.**
7. **Florisene – Excellent UK product produced by major pharmaceutical company.**
   http://www.florisene.com
   http://www.pharmacy2u.co.uk
   http://www.health4youonline.com

DIANA 35

Diana 35 is strictly a treatment for women and not for all women. Known medically as Cyproterone Acetate with Ethinyloestradiol, it is an oral contraceptive. It is often prescribed for severe cases of acne in women but has been found to halt androgenetic alopecia (female pattern baldness). Diana 35 is able to produce its results primarily because it is an anti-androgen properties. Success rates vary between 50 to 90 percent when used for periods of six months or longer. The higher figure obtained if the therapy is instigated during the initial symptom appearance. Diana 35 unlike Propecia does not specifically produce hair growth but allows undamaged hair follicles to return to a healthy state of production. If the follicles are undamaged healthy growth will occur and the surrounding scalp hairs thicken.

Diana 35 has long been a staple for combating female pattern baldness in Europe but has found slower acceptance in the United States. One beneficial side effect of this oral contraceptive is that it helps prevent osteoporosis

- **One interesting piece of research that relates to the use of contraceptives is that many of these medications contain copper. Too much copper in the body has been linked to hair loss. You can always check to see what is actually contained in your prescription. Be aware though the largest source of copper is also found in "hard" tap water. Simple blood tests can validate whether you are within the normal ranges that won't interfere with hair growth.**

SOURCES FOR DIANA 35

1.   **Diana 35 is best obtained by doctor's prescription. Always discuss with your prescribing physician any possible side effects you might encounter.**

YASMIN, DEMULEN, DESOGEN, ORTHOCYCLEN

These prescription drugs may not be recognizable to most men and probably only to a few women but they are estrogen dominant birth control pills. Even though oral contraceptives have long been linked to female hair loss these particular formulations are not. Quite the opposite hair loss specialists and doctors have found these particular medications flood the hair follicles with estrogen thereby reducing the testosterone linked to many cases of female pattern baldness. Plus if you're wondering this is the exact same DHT linked to male pattern baldness.

In regard to the prevention of female hair loss we suggest continuance of your present regime if you have found it to be satisfactory. Many women have long ago chosen a birth control method that is suitable for their body's chemistry. We only introduce this as an option.

•   **There have been recent user warnings about Yasmin so remember to consult with your doctor about possible side effects.**

SOURCES FOR YASMIN, DEMULEN, DESOGEN, ORTHOCYCLEN

1.   **Doctor's prescription**

ALFATRADIOL

This particular compound is the active ingredient found in the hair loss product known as Pantostin. Recognized more as a hair loss inhibitor as compared to hair growth agent its primary mechanism of action is insulation of the hair follicle from the effects of DHT. Even though many feel it is one of the weaker DHT inhibitors it has two qualities that distinguish it from many of the competitors. First it is almost totally free of side effects and two it is an excellent companion for the product Rogaine. The reason being is it allows minoxidil users to discontinue usage of that product once maximum results are attained. At that point you can keep the new hair created by the Rogaine with just a daily dosage of the Pantostin. The only caveat being that Pantostin is primarily found only in Germany. It does have a wide following among women in that country because of its ease of application and safety.

SOURCES FOR ALFATRADIOL

1. **Avixis - Pantostin**
    http://www.apotheke-online-internet.de
    http://www.mycare.de
    http://www.shop-apotheke.com
    http://avixis.com.mx
2. **Estradiol Valerate – Similar product 10 times more potent than Alfatradiol.**

SOAPWORT

Soapwort is a plant that contains saponins which are naturally occurring surfactants or detergents. The obvious advantage of these type detergents is they are less stressful to the scalp and skin and are naturally derived. The disadvantage though is most man-made ingredients now surpass these plants in cleansing ability, so soapwort is typically confined to usage as a foaming agent. What's interesting about the plant are its unique antibacterial properties that lessen the immune response when applied to the scalp. Because of this there is a notable reduction in hair loss. Though definitely linked to eradicating hair fall out, due to genetic baldness, widespread use of this ingredient we will always remain small because of the mentioned disadvantages.

SOURCES FOR SOAPWORT

1. **Kirk's Natural Shampoos and Conditioners**
    http://www.vitacost.com
    http://www.swansonvitamins.com
2. **Apivita Propoline Shampoo for Men and Women**
    http://www.apivita.com
    http://skincarerx.com
    http://www.softsurroundings.com

RED CLOVER

Red Clover is another supplement containing phytoestrogens that quite a few women have found helpful for combating hair loss. For years the oil of this plant has been prized for the treatment of psoriasis. The active ingredient being methyl salicylate. Australian research has deemed it as an effective suppressor of hot flashes and hair loss prevention agent for women.

This fairly cheap herb achieved its notoriety in the 1940's when herbal healer Harry Hoxsey proclaimed it as a cure for various cancers in women. His formula was popularly known as the "Red Clover Combination." Hoxsey at the time ran a chain of cancer clinics that used natural ingredients for the cure of this dreaded disease. His contentions were under continuous attack by the American Medical Association. The AMA maintained, at the time, the only legitimate cure for cancer was surgery and radiation. Hoxsey argued that these prescribed treatments of the AMA often resulted in lethal doses of radiation. Plus the surgery often severely disfigured women. Hoxsey for the largest part was labeled a quack. Later jailed, he withdrew to virtual seclusion.

Today many of the herbal solutions utilized by Hoxsey are widely recognized as having legitimate anti-cancer properties. Red Clover being one of them.

Red Clover though not as potent as soy, as a hair loss preventative, can alleviate the problem in many women.

SOURCES FOR RED CLOVER

1. **Walmart**
2. **Vitamin and Nutritional Stores**
3. **Alterna Caviar Clinical Daily Detoxifying Shampoo**
   http://www.sephora.com
   http://shop.alternahaircare.com
   http://www.fashionandbeautystore.com
4. **Nature's Way Red Clover**
   http://www.soap.com
5. **Puritan's Pride**
   http://www.puritan.com

IMAGING

One area that is about as controversial as it sounds is the use of imaging to grow hair. According to Doctor Gerald Epstein of the Mount Sinai Medical Center imaging to grow hair can work - if you do it actively enough.

To practice it Epstein suggests using the following strategy for twenty-one days at a time, then stopping for seven days. Then restart the same twenty-one day seven-day cycle until your hair begins to grow. Using this approach twice a day three minutes at a time is suggested.

IMAGING METHOD

To use. First make yourself comfortable and close your eyes. Now breathe in and out deeply three times as a warm sense of relaxation comes over you. Imagine yourself now being a gardener sensing, feeling, and seeing yourself plant new seeds for hair growth. See your scalp as a garden, ready to bring forth new life. Picture yourself walking through this garden with a bag of seeds made of growth hormones for the hair. The seeds are in the form of balls of golden light. Envision yourself seeding this fertile garden as you deposit to each follicle one of these golden balls from your hand.

Now water this whole area with golden water which you feel and sense as it is absorbed into the follicle and forms a golden network of fluids all through the scalp, as it nourishes each and every follicle causing it to grow. Breathe out. Visualize your hair as it begins sprouting upward through the scalp. Now breathe out one more time and open your eyes knowing new hair has begin to grow throughout your scalp.

Unbelievable as it may sound the mind is a very powerful vehicle. And if you think this idea is confined to "crackpots" think again. Proponents of imaging range from the most imminent physicians to top professional athletes. Many of these esteemed doctors claim imaging has shown its effectiveness for years in the healing process, by halting otherwise incurable diseases. Plus many professional athletes have acknowledged that just by constantly visualizing enhanced performance you can create optimal achievement. At worse the added relaxation is not going to hurt you.

Since imaging can vary with the individual you can enhance upon Doctor Epstein's approach to obtain the desired results. This method could possibly amaze you if you have the patience and imagination to use it. If you already have some knowledge of relaxation techniques you can add them to the regime to improve your results. It is not a requirement though.

TOPICAL CONCEALERS

Well before the development of any ingredient for hair loss concealers were put to use. These innovative wonders ranged from wigs to elaborate headgear to cloak the obvious. Literature abounds documenting the evolution of many of these devices for hiding hair loss.

Since results are never instantaneous in dealing with baldness it seems only fitting to include a couple of the more popular concealment methods. Concealers can be great for special occasions or when you feel you need that "added edge" in a social situation.

COUVRE

Probably the most recognized concealment offering in the hair loss marketplace is Couvre. This over the counter staple of the Hollywood stars and the quotably famous has many satisfied users. Combining a patented formulation with a variety of shades Couvre has allowed many people to gracefully blend away the bald. By matching an appropriate color type to your hair even some of the most trained eyes can be fooled into thinking you have more natural hair than you really do.

SOURCES FOR COUVRE

1. **Order forms in men's magazines such as Gentlemen's Quarterly.**
2. **Some of your local hair styling establishments.**
3. **Couvre and Dermatch sites**
    http://www.stylebell.com
    http://www.hairenvy.com
    http://www.dermatch.com

TOPPIK

Toppik is one of the newer commercially available concealers for those who suffer from hair loss. It is marketed by Spencer Forrest Incorporated. Toppik differentiates itself from its competition in that it is not a cream, cover up, or hair spray. Rather Toppik is composed of thousands of electrostatically magnetized micro fiber hairs that can instantly bond with the existing hairs on the scalp. By doing so a denser and fuller appearance is achieved on the scalp.

Application of Toppik is especially formulated for ease of use. By just shaking the scientifically designed molded container one can dispense the ultimate illusion of hair. And best of all it can withstand harsh weather, doesn't flake off on your pillow, won't stain, and can easily be washed out. Plus it's compatible with minoxidil. It's also available in a wide variety of colors that do include shades of gray. This product is of particular value if you have undergone hair transplants and desire to disguise the scalp trauma.

SOURCES FOR TOPPIK

1. http://www.toppik.com
   http://thickerhair.com

OTHER TOPICAL CONCEALERS

1. **Nanogen**
   http://www.nanogenhair.com
   http://www.onlyhairloss.com
2. **Hair So Real**
   http://www.hairlosstips.com
3. **GLH Hair Spray**
   http://www.salonweb.com
   http://hairloss101.com
4. **SureThik**
   http://surethik.com
5. **Caboki**
   http://www.caboki.com
6. **Fullmore**
   http://www.haircountry.com

STRUCTURED REGIME
HAIR GROWTH AND PREVENTION PROGRAM
(RECOMMENDATIONS)

SHAMPOO (CHOOSE ONE)

1. Therapro Shampoo
2. Nioxin Shampoo
3. Nizoral Shampoo 1% or 2%
4. Biotene H-24 Shampoo
5. Boost Super Stimulating Shampoo
6. Revita Shampoo
7. Jason Natural Biotin Shampoo
8. Nexus Biotin Shampoo
9. Jason Thin To Thick Shampoo
10. Herbal Glo Shampoo
11. Mill Creek Biotin Shampoo
12. Nano Shampoo *
13. Emu Oil Shampoo
14. Hair Fitness Shampoo
15. Spanish Garden Pepper Treatment Shampoo
16. Peter Lamas Chinese Herb Stimulating Shampoo
17. Markham Biotin Plus
18. Mont Source Moisturizing Shampoo
19. Sweet Sunnah Black Seed Oil and Henna Conditioning Shampoo
20. Tricomin Shampoo
21. Min (DHT Blocking) Shampoo for Thinning Hair

* The suggested use pattern for this product is twice weekly. Can be left on scalp for extended periods before rinsing to increase effectiveness. Should not be used on same day as Nano Conditioner.

CONDITIONER (CHOOSE ONE)

1. Thicker Hair Conditioner
2. Folicure Hair Conditioner
3. Biotene H-24 Hair Conditioner **
4. Nioxin Conditioner
5. Jason Thin To Thick Hair Conditioner
6. Nano Hair Conditioner***

7.   Emu Oil Conditioner
8.   Magick Botanicals Conditioner For Thinning Hair
9.   Herbal Glo Conditioner
10. Boost Super Stimulating Conditioner

** Many people rate Biotene H-24 as one of the better hair conditioners for hair loss.

*** The suggested use pattern of this product is twice a week. Should be used on alternating days if using Nano Shampoo. Can be left on scalp for extended periods before rinsing to increase potency.

SAW PALMETTO AND OTHER SUGGESTED VITAMINS

1.   Use tablet form of Saw Palmetto extracts. We strongly recommend Sundown Herbals Saw Palmetto Complex with Pygeum and Nettles. Similar European formulas cost hundreds of dollars.
2.   Use tablet forms of B-100 or B-50 containing Inositil, Choline, Biotin, PABA, or a good multiple vitamin containing these nutrients. Look for Zinc and Cysteine also.
3.   Solaray HAIRX
4.   Essential Fatty Acids
5.   MSM
6.   Soy Isoflavones
7.   Amino Acid Formula
8.   Ho Shou Wu (Fo-ti)

NEEM SHAMPOO, NIZORAL SHAMPOO, OR TAR SHAMPOOS

•   Suggested use pattern is twice a week for these products.

MINOXIDIL

•   Use the Minoxidil 2% or 5% formula nightly on the crown portion of the scalp after shampooing. Foam, cream, salve, and ointment formulations can be used on the frontal hairline. We also suggest using generic versions of minoxidil to reduce costs.

147

FOLLIGEN SPRAY SOLUTION OR LOTION

- Use on alternating days.
- Tricomin may also be used in place of Folligen.

PROSCAR OR PROPECIA

- Use as physician suggests. Refer to subject heading labeled Proscar.

SKINOREN OR FOLLIGEN CREAM

Skinoren or Folligen Cream are suggested for the frontal hairline. Either may be combined with 2% minoxidil. Used singularly, without minoxidil, Skinoren tends to have the better results in these areas of the scalp.

RETIN A

- Use as directed in article on Retin A. Should be used in tandem with 2% minoxidil or betamethasone.

OTHER PRODUCTS FOR CONSIDERATION IN YOUR PERSONAL PROGRAM

1. Thicker Fuller Hair Thickening Serum-Excellent for hair control.
2. Consort, Nioxin, and Roffler hair sprays-Not known for hair growth capabilities but excellent aroma.
3. Emu Oil
4. Recapture Hair
5. Green Tea Extracts
6. Nioxin Lift Volumizing Mist
7. Spectral DNC
8. Therapro Products
9. Grow Shampoo

PRECAUTIONS

With all of the suggested ingredients we suggest discontinuance if scalp irritation or redness becomes obvious. In the case of pharmaceutical or herbal agents for internal consumption we also recommend stoppage if side effects become noticeable or apparent. Following the prescribed directions for usage is always advisable. Data on some well-known ingredients for hair loss has not been included in these writings. The reasoning for this is that safe consumption has not been determined for these agents over extended periods of time. Furthermore most of these products will never be marketed for anything outside of their intended purpose.

One other caution we would especially like to give emphasis to is the overuse of vitamins, herbs, and nutrients. More is not necessarily better. We say this because there are a small percentage of people who "load up" on every ingredient they can put their hands on. This is very unwise and can often lead to side effects. We advise testing a few ingredients at a time at the suggested dosage. If after one to three months they appear to work for you continue with them. If not, discontinue and try some others. Just don't abuse it. Mega-dosing usually just creates a drain on your pocketbook.

RECEDING HAIRLINE TREATMENTS

To many the most traumatic effect of hair loss is the dreaded "M" hairline. Even though all of the ingredients have proven to be successful in treating frontal hair loss with time, some treatments are more successful at doing this than others. One particular treatment demonstrated to stimulate hair follicles in the frontal scalp areas is listed below. It is quick to apply regime, which should produce fine vellus hair on your forehead area within a month. If you are going to see thicker growth it should become apparent within four months. The ingredients you will need are:

- **Folligen Hair Growth Therapy Spray**
- **2% or 5% minoxidil solution**
- **Zinc formulation listed under that category.**

To use you should start the morning with about a 1/3-ml of 2% or 5% minoxidil applied to the areas of your scalp that have receded. Once this has dried lightly mist with the Folligen spray solution. One to two hours before you retire repeat the same application or replace the copper peptide solution with the zinc formula.

Other therapies that have also shown excellent results on the frontal hairline are the combination drugs of minoxidil plus Retin A or minoxidil plus Azelaic acid. With these combo therapies once a day usage on the frontal hairline has proven to be just as effective as twice a day. Remember minoxidil alone is effective on the crown portion of the scalp. The combo formulas on the other hand should only be utilized along the frontal hairline. Keeping this in mind the cost of this therapy can be reduced substantially.

For even more affordable solutions for the frontal hairline there are minoxidil 2% and 5% salves, gels, and ointments that can be found at Zooscape.

Another therapy that is receiving astounding reviews for its hair growth capabilities is a combination of betamethasone and Retin A. In fact a patent has been filed for this combination and hopefully we will see products combining these two ingredients shortly. What's exceedingly interesting is people have reported hair growth in as little as two days with most users reporting strong results within three weeks. Apparently Retin A is also capable of offsetting the skin thinning seen with overuse of betamethasone over extended periods of time. The compound is administered as a combination of betamethasone dipropionate 0.05% and tretinoin (retinoic acid) 0.0125%. Many pharmacists can readily compound this mixture for you by appropriately combing the creams. An additional suggested add-on to this treatment is emu oil shampoo. The biggest advantage of this therapy is that people have reported even with discontinuance the hair continued to grow and did not exhibit any shedding.

Plus let's not overlook Bimatoprost as a very potent treatment to regrow hair along the frontal hairline. It's expensive but the reported results tend to "stick" even when the medication is discontinued. More about this can be found under the appropriate heading.

Lesser known therapies therapy found to be effective for treating a receding hairline are cream versions of 2% Nizoral, MSM, and melatonin. The advantage of these treatments is they blend with the skin and can be left on the scalp for extended periods of time.

- **Remember to use the above solutions on the frontal hairline. Cheaper OTC minoxidil can be used in the crown areas.**

- **Many people have been well satisfied with minoxidil gels, salves, and ointments formulated for use on the frontal hairline.**

WHAT THEY DON'T TELL YOU CAN COST YOU
REDUCING YOUR PROPECIA COSTS

Ladies and Gentlemen one of the many things the hair loss gurus don't teach you is you can halt your hair loss for a lot less you can imagine with Propecia or Proscar otherwise known as Finasteride. What researchers don't tell you are these particular baldness treatments have a "flat line response" which is typical of many drugs. That probably doesn't tell you much until you understand what that translates to. Basically it means no matter how much of this medication you take to cure your hair loss the body only utilizes so much and discards the rest. In the case of Finasteride no matter what dosage you consume whether it is 5mg, 1mg, or .2 mg the body uses the exact same amount and the reduction in dihydotestosterone is identical for all dosages. In other words with all forms of commercially available Finasteride you will derive exactly the same benefits regardless of the size of the dosage. Using more in this case won't yield better results in fact it just means you consented to paying more money to grow hair.

Well astute people at this point might have picked up on the fact that if you can obtain the same results with any dosage why not utilize the most affordable route for growing hair, preventing pattern baldness, or just keeping the hair you already have. Well you can do just that by quartering Proscar then quartering it again or you can quarter the Propecia. In effect with one prescription of Propecia you can extend the benefits for up to four months by dividing the tablets.

Since all dosages of this popular hair loss drug effectively neutralize the existing DHT and it takes the body three or more days to synthesize newer DHT you can cut your costs even further. What studies have shown is many people can take any of these dosages every three days to stop a bald spot, curb a receding hairline, or even cure your thinning hair. The benefits were not dose dependant as long as you took the same dose at least every three days.

One of the biggest benefits of all that hasn't been mentioned is you can potentially lower your risk of side effects but that's no guarantee since all dosages accomplish exactly the same task.

Bottom line is with this particular hair loss medication you can obtain exactly the same results with a lower dosage used at least every three days. If you want to further reduce your costs just add a three-dollar pill splitter to your bill which can be purchased at any drugstore.

TIPS FOR THINNING HAIR

1. Do wash your hair on a daily basis. Amazingly the latest hair loss research indicates those who wash their hair at least three times a week are less likely to experience baldness. Most shampoos made today are mild enough to be used every day but watch out that it doesn't create an overly oily scalp. Washing your hair will give it a fuller appearance.

2. Do use conditioners. They increase the strength and elasticity of the hair shaft. Once a week in the case of short hair. Twice a week or more in the case of longer hair.

3. Avoid using inexpensive forms of vitamin E. Often times it contains estrogens that agitate hair loss. Dry and water-soluble mixtures are best.

4. Leave your hair short. This gives the scalp a fuller appearance and reduces stress upon the individual hair follicles when washing and brushing.

5. Thinning hair looks its best when trimmed on a monthly schedule.

6. Avoid excessive use of chocolates, alcohol, and OTC liquid antacids. These things have all been linked to hair loss. Most over the counter antacids are high in sodium.

7. Avoid excessive amounts of vitamins A and D. These nutrients may also contain large amounts of estrogens, dependent upon the source they are derived from. Even though they are essential for hair growth, too much of these supplements can cause side effects. Adequate amounts of these vitamins can be found in many green leafy vegetables and by exposing yourself to sunlight.

8. Do not over brush your hair. The myth that excessive brushing of the hair improves its health is just that, a

myth. If anything it places undo tension upon the scalp and can cause even greater hair loss.

9. Use brushes that don't pull on the hair. Purchase and use a hairbrush with bristles that don't scratch or injure the scalp.

10. Observe weight loss programs. Not eating a proper diet can cause hair loss.

11. Do drink eight glasses of fluids a day.

12. Use a good vitamin B-50 or B-100 product or one specifically formulated for the hair. It can and will enhance the condition of the hair and scalp in most people.

13. Massage your scalp periodically. This will stimulate blood flow to the hair follicles.

14. Don't continually over exercise. Cumulatively it can lead to calcium, potassium, zinc, and manganese loss. These nutrients are necessary for hair growth. Newer research indicates that more calcium and zinc is lost through sweating than once was thought.

15. Do get the proper amount of sleep based upon your needs. Research has shown that even small amounts of emotional stress can cause hair loss.

16. Don't have your hair over processed. But coloring normally doesn't affect hair loss unless it's overdone.

17. When coloring try a lighter tint than your normal hair's pigment. It makes bald spots less definable or noticeable.

18. Watch your salt intake. Swedish studies indicate that excess salt in the diet can result in hair loss.

19. Observe the medications that you take. Many prescription drugs definitely cause hair loss.

20. **If you use a part in your hair align it with the middle of your eye. Parts further to the side may accentuate baldness.**

21. **Watch the length of your sideburns. They can also draw attention to baldness.**

MEDICATIONS AND OTC DRUGS
THAT CAN CAUSE HAIR LOSS

While indeed genetics and many other factors play an important part in hair loss many OTC drugs and prescription medications can also encourage just the same. Due to the fact that many drugs can cause various bio-chemical changes in the body, to stimulate a healing or corrective process, it is not unusual that some medications exacerbate hair loss. Even though it is the goal of most manufacturers to continually lessen the side effects of medications it is not always possible to do so. Since re-establishing the health of a patient is always the first priority, often time's physiological changes that take place with various medications are ignored. This is especially true with regard to cardiac disease and chemotherapy. It is important to remember that once many of this conditions and disorders are brought under control hair loss will often diminish. Sometimes just an adjustment or change in the medication can lessen the hair loss. The critical thing is preserving the quality of the individual's life in all cases. Never discontinue a medication that can compromise your life or worsen a serious disorder.

When your doctor prescribes a medication it's also a good idea to ask if it will cause hair loss. Your doctor may not realize hair loss can be a side effect of the treatment. You can always ask him or her to check the Physician's Desk Reference which details the side effects of all prescription drugs. If the drug is linked to reversible alopecia, ask if another can be substituted. Even though some doctors may feel this can deal with an individual's vanity it is quite the opposite. Often times when an individual feels he looks better he feels better. Your pharmacist can also be an excellent source of information because that is their specialty.

Listed below are a few medications that may cause hair loss in some individuals.

CHOLESTEROL LOWERING DRUGS:

1. **Chofibrate (Atromis-S)**
2. **Gemfibrozil (Lopid)**

PARKINSON DISEASE MEDICATIONS:

1. Dopar
2. Larodopa

ANTICOAGULANTS:

1. Courmarin
2. Heparin

GOUT MEDICATIONS:

1. Loporin
2. Zyloprim

ANTIARTHRITICS:

1. Pencillamine
2. Auranofin (Ridaura)
3. Indomethacin (I\Indocin)
4. Napoxen (Naprosyn)
5. Sulindac (Clinoril)
6. Methotrexate (Folex)

EPILEPTIC DRUGS

1. Trimethadione (Tridione)

ANTIDEPRESSANTS

1. Various Tricyclics (Check Package Inserts)
2. Paxil
3. Prozac

BLOOD PRESSURE MEDICATIONS AND BETA BLOCKERS

1. Atenolol (Tenormin)
2. Metoprolol (Lopressor)
3. Nadolol (Corgard)
4. Propranolol (Inderal)
5. Timolol (Blocadren)

THYROID AGENTS

1. **Carbimazole**
2. **Iodine**
3. **Thiocyanate**
4. **Thiouracil**

BLOOD THINNERS, ANABOLIC STEROIDS

GLOSSARY OF TERMS

alopecia areata - A disorder of unknown origin characterized by sharply defined patches of sudden complete baldness. Sometimes referred to as "patchy baldness." Condition is more often temporary with limited damage to the hair follicles.

amino acids - organic acid containing amines (ammonia like chemicals). They link together in specific ways to form proteins and polypeptides.

anti-fungicidal - Ingredient or substance that inhibits the growth of a fungus.

antioxidant - A chemical that combines with free radicals that would otherwise attack molecules in the body, and abnormally oxidize them.

B-100 - Supplement or combination of vitamins that consist of all the B vitamins in 100 mg. or mcg. dosages. It preferably contains biotin, inositil, and choline.

cholesterol - A fat-soluble crystalline steroid alcohol found in animal fats, oils, egg yolks. It is widely distributed throughout the body. It is necessary for the synthesis of various steroid and sex hormones. There are basically two types of cholesterol the typical individual hears about. Those are cholesterol with high-density lipoproteins (HDL) and low density lipoproteins (LDL). The former being associated with increased life span and the latter with heart disease.

collagen - A connective tissue protein found in most parts of the body. Collagen loss as the result of aging leads to wrinkling of the skin.

crown galea - Thin membrane of skin found beneath the scalp and above the skull.

dermis - The dermis or corium is the inner layer of the skin. It contains the blood vessels, nerve endings, pigment cells, deposits of fat, sweat glands, oil glands, hairs, and muscle fibers.

dihydrotestosterone (DHT) - Hormone formed by the metabolism of the male hormone testosterone. Current research suggests DHT is the major causative component in male pattern baldness.

eczema - An inflammatory disease of the skin marked by itching, lesions, and a watery discharge.

enzyme - A protein which acts as a catalyst in metabolism. It is basically a substance that has the ability to accelerate or initiate chemical reactions in the human body.

epidermis - The epidermis is composed of the outer layer of the skin. There are five distinct layers composing this portion of the skin.

FDA - United States Food and Drug Administration.

free radicals - Substances thought to be related to the aging process and damage to the human body. Scavengers of these molecules such as antioxidants have been shown to lessen this damage or reverse it.

prostaglandin - Hormone like substances found in humans, which are necessary for many physiological functions to take place in the body.

hirsutism - Condition marked by sometimes profuse growth of hair on many parts of the body. Often times a side effect of a medication.

histamine - An amine released by a stressful condition being placed upon the body. It is necessary for growth and healing. It also widens the small blood vessels.

hydroxyl - A specific compound developed to retain moisture within the skin and slow the aging process.

Norwood Chart - Charting device displaying progressive stages of hair loss leading up to complete baldness.

OTC - Abbreviated term for "over the counter." In medical terminology it means a doctor's prescription is not required.

pitysporum - Fungus found chiefly on the scalp. Current research indicates it may have more of a relationship to dandruff than once was thought.

polyphenols - Naturally occurring substances found in plants that are high in antioxidants.

PSA Test - Medical test administered for the detection of prostate disease. Its accuracy is at about the seventy percent level.

psoriasis - Inflammatory condition of the skin with unknown origin. It is characterized by elevated irregularly shaped, patchy, reddish skin, with silvery scales. Normally it has little effect on the individual's overall health. Psoriasis can be extremely persistent but may subside with ordinary exposure to sunlight. Various agents such as tar and cortisone are used as treatment agents.

salicylates - Natural pain killing substances found in aspirin and aloe.

saturated - Fats containing no double or triple carbon bonds.

seborrhea - Inflammatory condition marked by over-activity of the sebaceous glands. Its appearance is usually confined to the upper portions of the chest and back but most often the scalp. This disorder can be identified by rounded red scaly patches which cause itching and scaling. It is often labeled profuse dandruff when found on the scalp. Identification of seborrhea can also be established by dissipation of the patches from the center outward, when clearing. It often "runs" the outline of the scalp.

sebum - Fatty lipoid substance emitted by the sebaceous glands.

testosterone 5-alpha reductase - Enzyme that converts testosterone into dihydrotestosterone (DHT) which makes the hair stop growing.

topical - Applied externally or to the outside, such as topical ointment.

unsaturated - Fats containing double or triple carbon bonds. May be more effective in reducing cholesterol.

vasodilator - Ability to cause dilation of a blood vessel.

GROWTH CYCLES OF HUMAN HAIR

An important part to understanding hair loss is being knowledgeable to the hair's growth cycles. These are the anagen, catagen, and telegon phases.

The anagen phase is the growing or active state of a follicle's life. Basically about eighty five percent of a typical scalp is in this stage. During this cycle reproductive cells create the bulb of the follicle, which in turn creates the shaft. Dependent upon the individual this stage can last from two to seven years.

In the catagen phase the hair has essentially stopped growing and is entering a resting period. This period can last up to six months. At one time many scientists thought this period was much shorter in length but the latest research tends to indicate otherwise.

In the final stage or telogen phase the hair has reached the end of its life cycle. This cycle also lasts about six months. At this point the hair is finally shed from the scalp and a new follicle begins forming in the pore. Dependent upon the abundance of hair and the length of these three cycles it is not unusual to see a loss of three hundred hairs a day in quite a few people. The average individual hair loss though is between one hundred and two hundred strands a day.

COMPOSITION OF HAIR

Under a microscope a hair cuticle will look somewhat similar to the scales on a fish. These scales are normally six to ten layers deep on a typical hair follicle. Their job is to protect the cortex, which lies directly beneath this. The cortex traps and holds sebum, which is the oily substance, secreted by the sebaceous glands. Sebum in effect makes the hair waterproof and increases the slip resistance of the hair. The direction of the scales on the cortex also allows water to drain more easily from the scalp. Hair that is damaged from chemicals, wind, sun or harsh treatment is often more porous because of the loss of these scales. Once damaged, the hair's water retention rate is increased. In addition, once these scales are lost the cortex can no longer protect itself with sebum therefore the brittleness factor is increased. This can lead to premature breakage and loss of hair.

The positive point to what we have been telling you about is that hair conditioners can eliminate most hair problems. Many conditioners employ sealants that can coat the hair shaft and thereby protect the cortex. Since the shaft is more penetrable when damaged, inversely, conditioning agents can be more readily absorbed. Many times chemically treated hair can actually look better than normal hair because of the superiority of these man-made ingredients. The caveat here is that undamaged hair as compared to damaged hair may experience a greater build-up from some of these excellent products. So beware. Regardless all conditioners and rinses do increase the slip factor which decreases breakage for all hair types.

HAIR CARE PRODUCT INGREDIENTS

What's in hair care products sold in today's marketplace makes for very stimulating conversation. The ingredients utilized range from the most basic elements to the more exotic botanicals. Theories on what is beneficial to the hair and the research behind it vary from manufacturer to manufacturer as much as the ingredients. Formulations are as bountiful as the products you view on the shelf. Remember though that price is not necessarily an indicator of quality. Many cheaper hair care products contain exactly the same ingredients as there more expensive rivals. The only true difference may be in the amount of cleansers used and the variations on the constituents employed. But the caveat here is that quite a few companies do manufacture products that are superior to others. It's just how much you're willing to pay for them and if you're astute enough to know the difference. Problems you may have with your hair or scalp may also only be eliminated by the use of certain ingredients. As one example in the case of dandruff, seborrhea, and psoriasis.

You should also be aware that every individual has different hair than the individual that may be standing right next to him. You may see similar color and types but that's about the extent of it. So quite the opposite of consumer gurus that advocate using dish washing detergent to clean your hair we take just the opposite view. Many hair care products do exactly what they claim to do, just not the same for everybody. The ingredients can be very helpful as long as you obtain enough of them.

INGREDIENTS

All hair care products manufactured in the United States are required by federal law to list ingredients utilized in descending order of quantity on the packaging. It is of particular importance to know what some of these compounds are since many scalps may be sensitive to some chemical constituents. What's good for one scalp may be completely antagonistic to another. The positive point though, in regard to allergic reactions, is that most sensitivities can be traced to the fragrance or coloring used in the product.

We will now list some of the more common ingredients found in hair care products so that that you can caution yourself if necessary. This knowledge base can also help you avoid paying too much for these toiletry items.

WATER

Water is the first ingredient listed on all products simply because it is the element of greatest quantity in all hair care products. The difference here is that some manufacturers do use purified or ionized water. This designation qualifies the liquid as free of minerals and other impurities that can build up on the hair. Water that has been purified is more suitable for blending with other substances, when the quantity of ingredients used is numerous. Unpurified water may contain enough iron, salt, chlorine, and fluoride that it renders some products almost worthless. Most manufacturers are aware of this so use of plain water is often limited to products that have a narrower list of ingredients.

DETERGENTS

Detergents are the cleansers of the hair and scalp. More often than not they are listed directly after water in quantity utilized on the packaging. Among chemists the word detergent is often used interchangeably when referring to surfactants. A surfactant is a long molecule that attaches one end of itself to oil and dirt and the other end to water, prior to being rinsed from the scalp. As one might assume there are strong detergents as well as milder ones. Often times a weaker detergent is combined with a stronger one to yield variations for dry, normal, and oily scalps. Some shampoos may contain as many as seven differing surfactants to establish the product's uniqueness and quality. The sudsing action that becomes visible when using these detergents is not directly related to their cleansing abilities. Some of the best surfactants produce few if any suds.

Listed below are some of the more common detergents or surfactants.

Sodium Lauryl Sulfate - Is one of the deeper cleansing high grade amonic surfactants.
Sodium Laureth Sulfate - Another of the amonic surfactants. Milder than lauryl sulftate. Most often used to offset harsher detergents.
Cocamide Dea - Mild detergent with antibacterial properties for sensitive scalps.

Other detergents found in this category are cocaidopropyl betaine, cocophodiacitate, ammonia lauryl sulfate, ammonia laureth sulfate, sodium cocoglercyl, and sodium lauryl sarcosinate. The coco's being high in fatty acids and the sodium blends helpful in removing dandruff flakes. It is important to point out that the ammonia bases detergents are milder and therefore better for sensitive scalps, but some individuals don't find them as effective at removing flakes on the scalp. So if you only lather up every two to three days it is best to use deeper cleansing detergents such as sodium lauryl sulfate.

LATHERING AGENTS

Lathering agents are present in shampoos chiefly because marketers have found people associate the cleansing ability of the shampoo with its lathering capabilities. The reality though is that lathering agents are just that and rarely indicate the true cleaning power of the product. To repeat what was mentioned in an earlier citation, some of the best detergents are low sudsing. But to convince people the detergents are working a lathering agent, more often than not, is added to the product.

Some compounds that create lather are cocamide mea, lauramide mea, lauric dea, and the Polysorbates. Of these the Polysorbates do possess good cleansing abilities in addition to their lathering capabilities.

QUATERNARY COMPOUNDS

Quaternary compounds or "quats", as they are often referred to, are chiefly the ammonia based ingredients found in hair care related products. They give hair a less sticky feeling and impart smoothness to it. This allows the hair to be brushed much more easily and the side benefit is a degree of shine. "Quats" are absolutely essential to having manageable hair. Various "quats" are used in both shampoos and conditioners. Typical quaternary compounds found in products are the ammonia based chlorides, behenalkonium betaine, bensalkonium chloride, quarternium 18 and 19, and stearalkonium chloride. In most cases the use of the word ammonia or chloride will designate a quaternary compound is being used in the product.

HUMECTANTS

These compounds attract water to the hair shaft thereby increasing the elasticity of the follicle. Some of the more common ones are glycerin, sorbitols, glycols, and the lipid groups. Some companies have developed sophisticated humectants that are patented and are only available to a limited number of manufacturers.

STABILIZERS AND PRESERVATIVES

These are ingredients that are purified and often pasteurized to stabilize other ingredients in the product. Many have antibacterial properties to ward off possible contamination. Some of the more popular ones are ascorbic acid, the parabens, and phenoxyethanol.

PROTEINS

Proteins can run the gamut from the most unimaginable to the clearly identifiable. They are used primarily to coat the cuticle to prevent it from becoming dry and brittle. Proteins give fine and thinning hair added fullness by thickening the cuticle. Some of the more expensive proteins have a moisturizing effect that can last for days. Often time you will see the word hydrolyzed used in conjunction with these compounds to identify smaller more absorbable fragments of protein. These minute pieces are better utilized by the cortex because of their size. Larger proteins are better for the cuticle in that they act more like sealants.

UREA

Urea allows ingredients in products to combine more effectively. It also serves to reduce the acidity of the product.

SILICONES

Silicones are substances that increase the slip resistance of the hair. By doing so static electricity and fly-away hair are substantially reduced. Typical silicones are dimethicone and cyclomethicone, which professedly bind to the hair better than any other ingredient. They do this by affixing themselves tightly to the cuticle and counteracting the effects of water. Doing so makes both these compounds excellent conditioners. The exception to this scenario being if your hair is already too oily or damaged. Use of these ingredients on these scalp types could give a somewhat greasy appearance to the hair. Many two in one shampoos utilize these ingredients.

AMINO ACIDS

Amino Acids act in much the same way as proteins. Coating the hair shaft or cuticle to prevent breakage and adding some moisture to the scalp. There are twenty-two known amino acids. They are sometimes labeled RNA or DNA on the packaging, if the individual acids have not been listed.

Listed below are the twenty-one of the known amino acids:

1. **Alanine**
2. **Aspartic Acid**
3. **Leucine**
4. **Iso-Leucine**
5. **Valine**
6. **Cysteine**
7. **Glutanic Acid**
8. **Glutamine**
9. **Histidine**
10. **Lysine**
11. **Methionine**
12. **Ornithine**
13. **Phenylalnine**
14. **Proline**
15. **Serine**
16. **Treonine**
17. **Cystine**
18. **Glycine**
19. **Tryptophan**
20. **Asparagine**
21. **Valine**

POLYMERS

Polymers are plastics that give the shaft additional thickness and strength. They are probably some of the few ingredients that can actually give the hair added shine. These ingredients will not injure your hair.

FATTY ACIDS AND ALCOHOL'S

These are compounds that prevent dehydration of the hair and scalp. Some of the better known ones are myristyl alcohol, stearyl alcohol, cetyl alcohol, oleic acid, palmetic acid, and stearic acid.

LANOLIN AND VARIOUS OILS

Oils typically offset the drying effects of detergents and various other ingredients used in the formulation itself. Every manufacturer utilizes oils to fashion the uniqueness of the product. These oils can range in price from the most expensive, to ones you can find in about every health and beauty aid encountered in the marketplace. The two most common types indicated on the packaging will be lanolin and petroleum gels. Other common types are mink oil, almond oil, wheat germ oil, mineral oil, jojoba oil, and even mom's old standby castor oil. If you analyze the various types of oils used in the formulations, the vast majority will either be vegetable or plant based. Most are meant to mimic the natural oil sebum secreted by our bodies.

ANTI-STATIC AGENTS

Anti-Statics are agents added to hair care products to reduce static electricity. By adding positive and negative ions, which attract to one another, the hair is made more manageable. Often this lack of control is referred to as the "frizzes" or fly-away hair. Typical anti-static agents are methylchloroisothiazolinone and methyllisothiazolinone.

FUTURE HAIR LOSS TREATMENTS

HISTOGEN

For years scientists have sought the silver bullet for hair loss and one such company now claims it may have the magic elixir for hair restoration. Enter the door Histogen HSC (Hair Stimulating Complex).

To give you some background Histogen is a biomedical company founded by Dr. Gale Naughton in 2007 that specializes in regenerative medicine. Through its research in culturing newborn cells in an embryonic environment and then deriving growth factors and Wnt proteins from this they developed an injectable proprietary formula for growing hair. This formulation was first tested in Honduras.

In the mentioned study 24 participants were chosen for a double blind placebo involved treatment regime. It involved a one time administration of an injectable form of Histogen. The patients scalp hairs were to be monitored for thickness, density, and hair count at appropriate points in time. At the end of the study (which was 12 weeks) all of the participants using Histogen experienced increases in all areas that were studied. Plus what was even more exciting was that all participants continued to show hair growth improvements a year later based upon a single injection. No evidence of any type of side effect was reported.

Histogen plans further development of its hair loss treatment in Singapore where it has received substantial foreign backing. They feel they will have a commercially viable product to be introduced in those areas by 2013. They hope to make the same available in the United States by the end of 2014.

ADDITIONAL TREATMENTS FOR YOUR CONSIDERATION

This section of our hair loss book contains a variety of the latest commercially available male and female baldness remedies that do not fall under the criteria of inexpensive solutions for hair loss. We include a short synopsis on each of these treatments because we felt some people might want to consider all options in combating their hair loss. Our presentation of the following should not be construed as an endorsement of any of these products. We advise investigating any of these treatments before purchase. Also certain well-publicized products and treatments are not listed because of an overall lack of satisfaction with customer service and with the accompanying results.

ADDITIONAL TREATMENTS GROUP A

ADENOGEN

Adenogen is a development of Shiseido a well-known Japanese cosmetic manufacturer. The chief ingredient is Adenosine which has been reported to have the same abilities as minoxidil. The manufacturers claim the product will increase the fullness of the scalp by stimulating its microcirculation. The product which can be used by both men and women should be applied twice daily and has no oily residue. The product is most often found at finer hair care salons and at upscale cosmetic counters.

SOURCES FOR ADENOGEN

1. http://www1.macys.com
2. http://www.usacosmetics.com
3. http://us.ozcosmetics.com
4. http://www.theevecare.com

ADVECIA

Advecia advertises itself as a dietary supplement to enhance the existing hair and as a hair loss preventative. The formula contains many well-known DHT blockers. What sets the product apart from the competition is the use of L-lysine and L-arginine. These particular amino acids have been shown to be particularly effective in halting hair loss and stimulating new hair growth. Other ingredients included in the formula are saw palmetto, green tree extract, beta sitosterol, grape seed extract, phytosterols, and procyanidins.

SOURCES FOR ADVECIA

1.   http://www.progressivehealth.com

AMERICAN CREW TRICHOLOGY HAIR RECOVERY SYSTEM

This is American Crew's three part system for men with thin hair. The various products include a shampoo rich in copper peptides, a concentrate with hops, and a patch that delivers the same ingredients as the concentrate. Predominantly a solution for thickening fine and thinning hair while at the same time encouraging robust growth of future hair. Seemingly this is a system for keeping the hair you have and making it less susceptible to breakage and other environmental damages. This company is also known for their revitalizing systems that also uses copper peptides. American Crew is known for high quality men's products.

SOURCES FOR AMERICAN CREW TRICHOLOGY HAIR RECOVERY SYSTEM

1.   http://hairloss.americancrew.com
2.   http://www.haircareusa.com
3.   http://www.sleekhair.com

AMINEXIL - DERCOS VICHY

The very well-known hair care company L'Oreal of France developed Dercos Vichy Aminexil. That being the case this is a hard product to ignore. The key ingredient is aminexil which prevents per follicular fibrosis. This is a condition that accompanies all forms of alopecia. Basically this is where the collagen around the hair root becomes rigid and tightens, pushing the root to the surface and causing premature hair loss.

Regular use of Dercos in a clinical placebo-controlled trial of 350 patients, demonstrated that patients using Dercos, over an 8 week period, had 8% hair re-growth, less hair loss, and experienced an increase in hair density of 6% compared to those who used a placebo.

The product lineup includes shampoos and conditioners which contain aminexil plus a more intensive routine composed of individual ampoules for daily use.

SOURCES FOR AMINEXIL - DERCOS VICHY

1. http://www.antiaging-systems.com
2. http://www.hairloss-hair-loss.com
3. http://www.frenchcosmeticsforless.com

ANCIENT SECRETS

Continuing with the theme of all natural ingredients are the 7Pe offerings from Ancient Secrets. This company's focus is on producing the best and safest hair growth products in the marketplace. Plus when we say all natural this company seemingly wrote the book on their usage. The lineup of products for all sexes and races include shampoos, conditioners, serums, and lotions. With a wealth of endorsements and competitive pricing it doesn't seem like you can go wrong here.

SOURCES FOR ANCIENT SECRETS

1. http://www.make-hair-grow-faster-7pe.com

ARCON TISANE

Arcon Tisane is a product with a twenty year history mainly sold in Europe. The makers make no extraordinary claims about the product except that it will stop anybody's hair loss. They don't say it will grow new hair on a bald scalp but if you're not too far along in the process you could see some good results. In other words this proprietary nutritional supplement will allow you to keep what you have, thicken the existing hair, and encourage new growth. The primary ingredient is Fenugreek which we fully endorse as a treatment for thinning hair. This herbal has been used since ancient times as potent remedy for hair loss.

The product line-up for males and females includes shampoos, conditioners, capsules, tinctures, and a silk serum. All of the products do contain the active ingredient Fenugreek. There is a new Arcone Plus formula which contains a greater array of trace minerals and vitamins. This is predominantly for people who might have some known deficiencies in these areas.

SOURCES FOR ARCON TISANE

1. http://www.arcontisane.com.au
2. http://www.arcon-international.de

AVACOR

Avacor has garnered much of its popularity from an aggressive marketing campaign seen quite often on TV. Now advertised as extra strength minoxidil (5%) the product line-up has lost much of its luster. Included products are a shampoo, conditioner, hair thickener, and multi-vitamin supplement that can be used by both men and women.

SOURCES FOR AVACOR

1. http://www.avacor.com

ADDITIONAL TREATMENTS GROUP B

BIOFEN

Biofen has probably been around the longest with regard to the sale of all natural herbal supplements for hair loss. They distinguish themselves in the marketplace by pointing out the fact that they utilize multiple dht inhibitors in their formulations. Also Biofen stresses their product is chiefly for hereditary androgenic alopecia (AGA).

Some of the active ingredients utilized are saw palmetto, fenugreek, and flax lignans. The product lineup includes the hair loss supplement plus shampoos and conditioners for both men and women.

SOURCES FOR BIOFEN

1. http://www.biofen.com

BIOSCAL AND BIOSCALIN

Bioscal and Bioscalin are products developed and tested at the University of Helsinki, Finland by Professor Kai Setala and Dr. Ilona Schreck-Purola. Bioscal is predominantly sold in the United States and

Bioscalin sold in Europe. The mentioned researchers are considered experts in the field of hair loss. The makers claim the formulas are the most effective and best documented non-pharmaceutical products sold in the world. The ingredient list is proprietary so it is difficult to compare the similarities to other solutions. Imitations of the formulas have often contained a healthy amount of Polysorbate 80. To be accurate though the makers claim these are the original formulations of the often imitated compounds.

The product line-ups for both men and women contain revitalizers, elixirs, concentrates, supplements, plus shampoos and conditioners.

SOURCES FOR BIOSCAL AND BIOSCALIN

1.   http://www.hairgrowthpartner.com

ADDITIONAL TREATMENTS GROUP C

CELLEX-C

Cellex-C is a niche product with one intended purpose. It is meant for hair loss related to pregnancy. Plus this is no small market segment it's almost gigantic. The formula itself combines natural sugar polymers with plant-derived phyto-chemicals and essential amino-acids to help control post-partum alopecia (hair loss). Immediately after usage the naturally derived glycosaminoglycans should impart a greater fullness to the scalp which should lift the spirits of many women during this trying time. Though not prescribed for long term usage it fits the bill for an unfilled section of the hair loss market

SOURCES FOR CELLEX-C

1.   http://www.cellex-cjunior.com
2.   http://www.perfumezilla.com

CLAIR'S HAIR TREATMENT

Clair's Hair Treatment seemingly started out as home based business that expanded to E-Bay and later on to its own World Wide Web sites. The product for men and women is fairly cheap. The chief ingredient is a topical version of saw palmetto combined with twelve other herbals. Some of these constituents are aloe vera, nettle leaf extract, gingko biloba, and thyme extract. There are many anecdotal comments on these web sites testifying to the effectiveness of the product but no real research to support the claims. The redeeming feature though is if ineffective at least it didn't cost a fortune to find out it doesn't work.

SOURCES FOR CLAIR'S HAIR TREATMENT

1.   http://www.clairshairtreatment.com

CORVINEX

Corvinex produces an array of products for men and women but is chiefly known for its hair loss supplement. Basically a vitamin, mineral, amino acids, and herbal formula it contains about every conceivable thing for fighting hair loss you could want. The follicle spray, shampoos, and hair conditioners likewise contain an array of ingredients that rival and exceed some of the better known names in the hair loss industry.

SOURCES FOR CORVINEX

1.   http://www.corvinex.com

CRE-C SHAMPOO

Cre-C shampoo is a product of Mexico with a considerable following on E-Bay. Other than the fact that the product contains all natural ingredients there doesn't seem to be an abundance of known hair growth stimulants in it. Then again the product has evolved from an age old formula of the Tepoztecan Indians long noted for beautiful hair. The shampoo which can be used by men and women lists lemon essence, nettle, aloe vera, verbain, jojoba, espinosilla, and chamomile as some of its primary ingredients. The makers claim the shampoo literally floods the follicle with an abundance of natural herbals that in turn halt hair loss. Many people report a noticeable decline in hair loss and increase in thickness of their hair within 1-3 months usage. People also report the shampoo must be shaken well to fully distribute the ingredients before shampooing. Plus since it is all natural and doesn't contain the harsher detergents most of us are familiar with other users have reported the hair feeling less clean. Undoubtedly some of this can be explained by the all botanical nature of this formulary.

SOURCES FOR CRE-C SHAMPOO

1. http://www.justbeautysupplies.com
2. http://www.ebay.com

CRINAGEN

Crinagen is a product developed by Doctor Nasser Razack. The active ingredients are ginkgo biloba, saw palmetto, niacin, vitamin B6, and zinc acetate. This product has long been a staple of the hair loss product industry. Doctor's Razack's newest product is Natrecia which is vitamin, mineral, and herbal supplement meant to treat both benign prostatic hyperplasia and androgenic alopecia. This product is similar to many that are used to treat BPH but it does have an attractive price when purchased in quantity.

SOURCES FOR CRINAGEN

1. http://www.raztec.com

CURETAGE

Curetage markets a line of hair loss products that distinguish themselves in the marketplace by utilizing a long list of all-natural ingredients and botanicals. The product lineup for men and women is composed of cleansers, conditioners, scalp purifiers and revitalizers, plus their root stimulator. The root stimulator, which is the centerpiece of their therapy, is an intensive leave-in scalp treatment for all hair types. Overall it is considered a very good hair care treatment system for all stages of thinning hair.

SOURCES FOR CURETAGE

1. http://www.curetage.com

ADDITIONAL TREATMENTS GROUP D

DEAD SEA ANTI-HAIR LOSS PRODUCTS

Premier hair loss products were developed after their research indicated balding may be the result of sodium accumulation in the hair follicle. This buildup of sodium may be the result of stress, environmental reasons, malnutrition, or hereditary factors. Normally a fat gland within the follicles aids in the regrowth of hair and lubricates the scalp against dryness and bacteria but with male and female pattern baldness it becomes clogged thereby preventing normal hair growth. To offset these maladies formulations were conceived to dissolve the accrual of debris blocking the follicle. The product line-up can be used by both men and women and includes shampoos and conditioners. Some of the listed ingredients are a blend of Dead Sea minerals, keratin, ginger, garlic, and gentian.

SOURCES FOR DEAD SEA ANTI-HAIR LOSS PRODUCTS

1. **http://deadseaserum.com**
2. **http://premier-beautycare.com**

DERMENODEX

Dermenodex is one of a few formulations, besides Shiseido's Adenogen, containing the active ingredient Adenosine which is as effective as minoxidil without the safety concerns. It is marketed by American Beauty Supply, makers of the Sedu and Solia line of hair care products. The theory behind Adenosine is based upon enhancing microcirculation within the scalp to encourage optimal hair growth. The formulations include serums, shampoos, and conditioners. Unfortunately products containing this excellent ingredient have fallen victim to the competition.

SOURCES FOR DERMENODEX

1. **http://www.folica.com**

DOCTOR LEWENBERG'S FORMULA

Doctor Lewenberg is truly one of the pioneers in developing products that use a combination of minoxidil and Retin-A to combat male and female hair loss. Through extensive study he has developed a two phase program to first grow hair then a maintenance step to provide optimal results for the hair growth you've already experienced. These products are patented and have a strong following. Though considered pricey it is a well-established line of products.

SOURCES FOR DOCTOR LEWENBERG'S FORMULA

1.   http://www.baldspot.com

ADDITIONAL TREATMENTS GROUP E

EUCAPIL – FLURIDIL

Eucapil is a cosmetic product approved for the treatment of androgenetic alopecia in the European Union. As yet it has not been approved for marketing in the United States even though the product promotes itself as having no known systemic absorption. Biophysica Incorporated of San Diego though developed the product in the United States.

The theory behind the product is it counter-effects the changes seen within the hair follicle common with female and male pattern baldness. With repeated usage the makers claim your hair will take on added fullness and a healthier appearance.

SOURCES FOR EUCAPIL – FLURIDIL

1.   http://www.eucapil.com
2.   http://www.eucapil-shop.eu

EXO BALANCE

A relatively new product to the marketplace Exo Balance Hair Regrowth Solution is advertised as an all-natural non-prescription formula for both stopping hair loss and aiding hair regrowth in both men and women. The solution itself is designed to enhance the circulation of the scalp while at the same time correcting for the loss of moisture, flora, and nutrients found within the follicle. These particular conditions thought to be attributable to the environmental plus chemical and hormonal changes within the body. The main ingredient of this product Vitaliste is a combination of plant derived substances developed to counteract these particular scalp imbalances. The company claims that with as little as eight week's usage the solutions can double the diameter of the existing hair. Primary means of research for this product have been conducted with electron microscopes.

SOURCES FOR EXO BALANCE

1.   http://www.exobalance.com

ADDITIONAL TREATMENTS GROUP F-G

FABAO

Fabao is a product developed by Doctor Zhang-Guang Zhao, who is considered to be one the leading international experts on thinning hair. His formulas enjoy one of the longest reputations for commercially available hair loss products in the world. The original formula Fabao 101-D is chiefly known for utilizing capsicum as a hair growth ingredient.

SOURCES FOR FABAO

1.   http://www.fabao.com

FERM T SUPER HAIR ENERGIZER

Ferm-T Super Hair Energizer utilizes an exclusive solution composed of twenty different botanicals plus jojoba oil. The makers of this product claim their special development and aging process initiates a healthy scalp enabling hair restoration. The product accomplishes this feat by clearing the scalp of excess sebum that has plugged the pores inhibiting proper growth of the hair. As many people know jojoba oil has long been suggested as a cure for pattern baldness and the longevity of this product in the marketplace suggests it is a viable option for treating your hair loss problems.

SOURCES FOR FERM T SUPER HAIR ENERGIZER

1.   http://www.superhairenergizer.net

FNS OSMOTICS FOLLICLE NUTRIENT SERUM

FNS Osmotics Follicle Nutrient Serum was at one time named Pileil, which was breakthrough product developed by Israeli scientist Dr. Ella Lindenbaum. Initial testing showed the product was almost a medical marvel because it grew hair with about every tested subject. Further testing though was abruptly halted and the original formulation was then sold to Osmotics. Speculation was the formula could be so easily duplicated that it would lose much of its financial value if not passed along to a manufacturer. Though still a proprietary formula the listed ingredients are mainly a mixture of vitamins, minerals, and amino acids. The product lineup for males and females includes revitalizing shampoos and conditioners plus the nutrient serum.

SOURCES FOR FNS OSMOTICS FOLLICLE NUTRIENT SERUM

1.   http://www.osmotics.com

ADDITIONAL TREATMENTS GROUP H

HAIR CUBED

Hair Cubed in their own words is a concoction of organic microfibers that attach to the surrounding hair giving the scalp a fuller appearance. Sold in eleven different colors to blend with your natural hair its chief advantage seems to be in the delivery method which is a spray. Competing products seemingly use a salt shaker approach for administering their particular blend of fibers.

SOURCES FOR HAIR CUBED

1.   http://www.haircubed.com

HAIR GENESIS

Hair Genesis is a well-respected company in the hair loss industry that markets a proprietary group of hair loss products chiefly derived from botanicals. The product lineup for men and women include shampoos, conditioners, vitamins with known dht blockers, and a topical activator serum whose ingredients are listed below. Hair Genesis is a leader in testing and research with regard to it hair loss system and ingredients.

Ingredients included in Hair Genesis topical activator serum: isopropyl alcohol, oleic acid, LSESr 85/95% liposterolic content (saw palmetto extract), lauric acid, palmetic acid, beta-sitosterol, stigmasterol, cycloartenol, lupeol, lupenone, 24-methyl-cycloartenol, oligomeric proantho-cyanidin, oleth-20, evening primrose oil, genestein, pygeum africana extract, Japanese green tea extract, GLA, borage oil, macadamia nut oil, propylene glycol, nonoxynol 10, polysorbate 80, camellia sinesis extract, biotin.

SOURCES FOR HAIR GENESIS

1.   http://www.hairgenesis.net

HAIR GROWTH LASER

Marketing themselves as a better and more cost effective alternative to the current crop of hand held laser brushes this product seems like a winner in many respects. What you get with this device is a commercial quality free standing laser unit that offers full coverage for the affected areas of the scalp. It can be used by both men and women. Adding to the convenience is your ability to sit and relax while receiving your laser treatment. The suggested usage is three times a week for twenty minute periods. Offered at a price of $549 this might indeed be one of the better bargains in hair loss control without all the work of hand held units.

SOURCES FOR HAIR GROWTH LASER

1.   http://www.femalehairlaser.com
2.   http://www.50lasers.com

HAIR PRIME

Hair Prime promotes itself as an all-natural alternative to Propecia and Rogaine that provides a healthier environment for hair to grow. The makers consider this to be a more ethical manner in which to advertise their product. The treatment system for both sexes includes a shampoo to prepare the scalp for application of the Hair Prime lotion, which combats the effects of DHT on the scalp. Additional parts of the regime include a herbal and multi-vitamin supplement plus a scalp primer to further protect the scalp from cosmetic and environmental damages.

SOURCES FOR HAIR PRIME

1.   http://www.unibio.com

HAIR SIGNALS

From the makers of Folligen comes their newest product Hair Signals. What's unique about this formula is it contains even more DHT blockers and growth enhancers than the original version. Skin Biology claims this new combination of ingredients act in a synergetic fashion to both halt hair loss and create new hair growth. Some of the ingredients utilized are, saw palmetto, beta sitosterol, Polysorbate 80, pygeum, and tea extracts. Copper peptides are also included. The product mix comes in a lotion and cream version. The lotion is meant to be applied over the entire scalp whereas the cream is for more targeted therapy such as the frontal hairline.

SOURCES FOR HAIR SIGNALS

1. http://www.onlyhairloss.com
2. http://www.salonweb.com

HAIR STIMULATOR

Hair Stimulator markets itself as an American company selling all natural all organically formulated hair loss products for men and women. The buzz phrase here is being no artificial ingredients. What's unique about HLPC products is within the past few years many leading hair care specialists now claim the best way to keep you hair is to go the all-natural route as put forth by this company. The chief active ingredient in most of this line-up of shampoos, conditioners, lotions, and vitamins is saw palmetto. One of their centerpiece products is the Daily Stimulator Plus with Minoxidil which is a lotion that can be applied once daily. Pricing is not steep.

SOURCRES FOR HAIR STIMULATOR

1. http://shop.hlpcproducts.com

HAIR-TEK HAIR BUILDING FIBERS

Hair-Tek emerges from a large group of products that specialize in bonding keratin hair fibers to the scalp to give it a fuller appearance. Product is available in seven different colors for men and women.

SOURCES FOR HAIR-TEK HAIR BUILDING FIBERS

1.   http://www.hair-tek.com

HAR VOKSE

Har Vokse markets a two part system for dealing with your hair loss. Included with it are a supplement and regrowth spray. The products themselves are very similar to Viviscal and incorporate marine polysaccharides as the primary ingredient. Other ingredients found in the formulations include amino acids, zinc gluconate, grape seed extracts, vitamin B complex, green coffee extracts, chlorophyll, the B-Complex, plus vitamins C&E.

SOURCES FOR HAR VOKSE

1.   http://www.harvokse.com
2.   http://buyharvokse.org

HERBAL ESSENTIALS

Herbal Essentials distributes a group of botanical based hair loss products for men (Hair Regain) and women (Hair Renew) that will likely become better known in the future. The reason being is that recent tests have shown that one of their primary ingredients, which is saw palmetto, is indeed an effective hair loss preventive and hair growth ingredient in topically applied formulations. Adding to that list are other effective dht blockers plus capsicum. The latter also being a potent hair growth stimulant. Both of Herbal Essentials systems include shampoos and conditioners.

SOURCES FOR HERBAL ESSENTIALS PRODUCTS

1.   http://www.endhairlossnaturally.com

HERBAL H

Herbal H Advanced Hair Growth Formula is one of the many variants of minoxidil combining botanicals and herbs to achieve greater delivery into the hair follicle. In this case the ingredients found in the formula, besides the 2% minoxidil, are maima, ginseng, angelica, saw palmetto, and polygonum mutiflorum. The makers claim what distinguishes their product from others is their "Penetrating Peel Technology." According to the developers this clears the follicle of excess sebum and debris allowing for new hair growth in as little as thirty days. Full results can be seen in about three months. The makers also say you can discontinue usage, except for routine maintenance, once you achieve the desired results.

Since newer versions of minoxidil now utilize advanced nano and liposome delivery systems whether this type system is as promising as it once was is up to debate.

SOURCES FOR HERBAL H

1.   http://www.herbal-h.com

HLCC SCRIPTS

HLLC Scripts is the total one-stop Internet stop for all your hair loss needs. This online shop sells complete hair loss treatment programs for the individual who wants to shop discreetly or purchase it all from one business. The product line ups for both men and women include shampoos, conditioners, laser brushes, topical concealers, and even with specially formulated versions of minoxidil. If you want it they likely have it. Not cheap but highly recommended.

SOURCES FOR HLCC SCRIPTS

1.   http://www.wheredidmyhairgo.com

ADDITIONAL TREATMENTS GROUP I

INNEOV HAIR MASS

This is a particular product we are extremely enthusiastic about but due to its price and availability it finds its way into our group of additional hair loss products for your consideration. The big plus of this product is L'Oreal of Paris developed it. L'Oreal has a worldwide reputation for quality hair care products.

The product itself is sold as a nutritional supplement used twice daily. The chief ingredients are taurine (150 mg.), green tree extract (145 mg.), zinc (15 mg.), and a small amount of grape seed extract. All of these ingredients are included in our groups of inexpensive ingredients so you can always develop your own regime based upon that.

Taurine alone is considered one of the better supplements for hair loss and is currently enjoying quite a reputation for its anti-aging effects upon the body. It has no known side effects. Zinc as always is still one of the most under-estimated minerals for igniting new hair growth and inhibiting further loss of hair. Used in combination L'Oreal asserts these ingredients have a synergetic effect deep within the root of the follicle that will continuously boost the growth of thick, dense, and glossy hair. Since again this is a nutritional supplement these ingredients are also beneficial to the heart and liver.

SOURCES FOR INNEOV HAIR MASS

1. http://www.parafarmacia-online.com
2. http://www.dermthings.com

ADDITIONAL TREATMENTS GROUP J

JUST NATURAL ORGANIC CARE

As the title exemplifies this is a group of hair loss products containing a robust lineup of all natural ingredients. As research has indicated many of the traditional additives utilized in hair care products may be the root cause of most thinning hair. In affect these formulations from Just Natural Organic depart from the traditional route of harsh cleansers and chemicals that can irritate the scalp causing more harm than good. So if you're looking for an array of products devoid of annoyances that may agitate sensitive scalps you can purchase your hair care regime here.

SOURCES FOR JUST NATURAL ORGANIC CARE

1. http://www.justnaturalskincare.com

JUVELINE

Juveline is a product developed by Elsom Research specifically for receding hairlines. The formulation utilizes microscopic nanosphere technology as the delivery system for an array of various vitamins and botanicals into the frontal hairline. The ingredient list is a long one but contains an ample supply of Vitamins A, C, and E. Other components of the product are nettle root, pygeum bark, smilax root, and desert cacti extracts. Included with that are MSM, arginine, zinc oxide, niacin, menthol, and copper chloride. The whole delivery process of these components though is dependent upon phosphatidylcholine and cyclodextrin. The former being one of the most advanced anti-aging ingredients known and the latter facilitating nano encapsulation. As you can probably guess this is not one of the cheapest products to be found for hair loss.

SOURCES FOR JUVELINE

1.   http://www.elsomresearch.com

ADDITIONAL TREATMENTS GROUP K

KERACYTE-B

One thing there can be no argument about is this product has a hefty price tag. On the plus side Keracyte-b claims it has the world's most advanced hair care formula. The makers of this product, Derma Plus, believe they have found the answer to hair loss and graying hair by creating a synthetic type keratin called Elastatropin (Tropoelastin). Elastatropin in essence helps restore the natural elastin content in scalp that is lost throughout the aging process. Even though this product is a marvel of modern science, few people have reported positive results. Perhaps with a more reasonable price tag the answers to whether this is a great product or not will finally be unlocked.

SOURCES FOR KERACYTE-B

1.   http://www.keracyte.com

KERATASE DENSIFIQUE (L'OREAL)

Keratase Densifique is the latest and probably the most astounding offering from the laboratories of Recherche Avance L'Oreal. Touted as the first method for awakening dormant hair on actual bald scalps it is causing quite a stir world-wide. Unlike many companies that concentrated on stem cell implants to induce hair growth L'Oreal committed its resources to finding natural treatments that could stimulate these particular cells into once again reproducing. Out of this came Densifique whose active ingredient is stemoxydine with a combination of B vitamins. This particular compound literally floods the follicle with oxygen and stimulates the stem cells to once again regrow hair. In testing with 101 subjects an overall increase of 4% in scalp density was observed over a three month period. This basically transfers to an increase in hair counts of 1500 hairs. The caveat here though is the high price and whether the hair continues to grow. L'Oreal has not been totally specific with these concerns but company literature indicates the treatment is only needed daily for three months. Based upon the fact that is a topically applied treatment with few side effects the comparative yearly costs between it and some hair loss pharmaceuticals might be equal.

SOURCES FOR KERATASE DENSIFIQUE

1. **Can be found at large US internet resellers and throughout Europe.**

KERIUM ANTI-HAIR LOSS TREATMENT

Kerium is a formulation developed by La Roche Posay a well-known manufacturer of skin care products. The theory behind these offerings, similar to that of Revlon's, is that hair loss is precipitated by multiple stress factors. In the case of men most of these causative agents are present year round where with women they can be cyclical in nature such as the case of hormones. To La Roche Posay pattern hair loss is triggered when the body feels a stress factor placed upon it. That in turn sets off micro-irritation in the scalp, which transfers directly to the hair bulb. Once this occurs it triggers a hair loss phase. To compensate for these things dermatologists at La Roche Posay developed a breakthrough ingredient that counteracted an essential acceleration factor they had observed in male and female pattern hair loss. This particular agent they developed being madecassoside which reabsorbed the mentioned micro-irritation thereby preventing the chain reaction in the follicle that triggers hair loss.

The product lineup for both men and women contains the serum, gels, shampoos, and conditioners.

SOURCES FOR KERIUM ANTI-HAIR LOSS TREATMENT

1.   http://parfumsetbeaute.com
2.   http://www.pharmamundi.com

KEVIS

Kevis is probably one of the better-known hair loss products in many parts of the world. Their product formulations address hair loss and scalp hygiene through the application of the biological compound hyaluronic acid. Plus this is a specially patented formula of hyaluronic acid. Product research and testing is some of the most thorough in the industry. The product lineup for both men and women is an extensive one and sales are chiefly made by phone consultation.

• **Kevis was acquired by More Naturally, Inc. a company known for the use of natural ingredients. Kevis products will remain the same just with new labeling.**

SOURCES FOR KEVIS

1.   http://www.morehairnaturally.com

KORRES MEN MAGNESIUM & WHEAT PROTEINS ANTI HAIR LOSS SHAMPOO

Korres is a well-known name in all natural hair care products. With their clinically tested hair loss shampoo and lotion they've again created another unique combination. This particular lineup is based upon combining wheat proteins, calcium, magnesium, manganese, zinc, and vitamin B-5 to curb men's hair loss and create new hair growth. In addition these ingredients substantially increase the natural elasticity of the hair and prevent premature breakage extending the life expectancy of the present hair.

SOURCES FOR KORRES MEN MAGNESIUM & WHEAT PROTEINS ANTI HAIR LOSS SHAMPOO

1.   http://www.lookfantastic.com
2.   http://www.lookmantastic.com
3.   http://www.bathandunwind.com

ADDITIONAL TREATMENTS GROUP L

LACINIA HAIR LOSS LOTION

Lacinia Hair Loss Lotion for males and females is one of the few products utilizing topically applied green tea (EGCG) as the active ingredient. Even though green tea is an established hair growth stimulant and hair loss preventative it is most often utilized in liquid or supplemental forms. Lacinia claims their formula can arrest and grow hair within a week with the vast majority seeing obvious results in six to eight weeks. Other ingredients found in the lotion are biotin, inositil, and zinc oxide.

SOURCES FOR LACINIA HAIR LOSS LOTION

1.   http://www.lacinia.com
2.   http://www.conceptcosmetic.com

LANADIL

Lanadil was a hair loss system specifically created for women but now includes products for men. What makes the products unique is a timed-release non-alcohol based nanosphere delivery mechanism for minoxidil. The makers claim this patented process allows for deeper penetration into the follicle which in turn creates greater hair growth. These nanospheres which are less than 100nm in size allow for the depositing of pure bioactive minoxidil deep within the hair bulb. The product lineup includes a shampoo, conditioner, and the treatment. Not a cheap system it does offer a delivery system for minoxidil without the usual irritating scalp itch and drying effects of the OTC alcohol propylene glycol based products.

SOURCES FOR LANADIL

1.   http://www.lanadil.com

LASER COMB

Sales for the laser comb skyrocketed when the United States Food and Drug Administration gave its approval to the technology. The principle behind it is low level light emitting lasers stimulate circulation and cellular metabolism which in turn stimulates hair growth as long as there is a viable follicle. There are now many versions of the laser comb and it is wise to examine the many offerings because of the current costs involved.

SOURCES FOR LASER COMB

1. http://www.hairmax.com

LEONOR GREYL HAIR LOSS PRODUCTS

Leonor Greyl is one of the many European companies that base their approach upon the idea that DHT is not the common culprit behind most hair loss. This lineup that is exclusively for women contains some of the finer hair care products to be found. The problem though is many of these formulations can be found at cheaper prices with some of the exact ingredients. The attention though to the particular formulations responsive to female hair loss though is undeniable.

SOURCES FOR LEONOR GREYL HAIR LOSS PRODUCTS

1. http://www.leonorgreyl.com
2. http://www.leonorgreyl-usa.com

ADDITIONAL TREATMENTS GROUP M

MELANCOR

Melancor is unique in that it one of the few products created specifically to rejuvenate your natural hair color. Advertised as a totally safe method to blend away your gray hair this twice a day pill is truly enticing. The proprietary formula contains ingredients that have been linked to curbing hair loss also.

SOURCES FOR MELANCOR

1. http://www.melancor.com

MINOXIDIL MAX

Without question one of the ultimate sites to be visited for affordable and varied versions of the hair loss medication minoxidil is

Minoxidil Max. Many of the products are formulated to reduce the irritations and side effects of this well-known product. The product line-up includes:

1. Lipogaine - An exclusive and trademarked combination of 5% minoxidil, procyanidin oligomers, 5% azelaic acid, saw palmetto extract, beta-sitosterol, gamma and alpha linolenic acids, plus oleic acid with a liposome delivery.
2. DualGen15 - Contains 15% minoxidil with 5% azelaic acid.
3. DualGen10 - Contains 10% minoxidil with 5% azelaic acid.
4. DualGen 5 - Contains 5% minoxidil with 5% azelaic acid.
5. DualGen 5 without Propylene Glycol- Contains 5% minoxidil with 5% azelaic acid.
6. EssenGen 15 - 15% minoxidil.
7. EssenGen 5 - 5% minoxidil without propylene glycol.
8. EssenGen 2 - 2% minoxidil for women.
9. Minoxidil strength testing kit.

SOURCES FOR MINOXIDIL MAX

1. http://www.solutions4hairloss.com
2. http://www.minoxidil4hairloss.com
3. http://minoxidilmax.com

MTS HAIR RESTORATION COMPLEX

MTS (Microneedle Therapy System) is a company that has sunk its full teeth into scalp roller technology for renewing the scalp and battling hair loss. Its hair restoration lineup includes a patented scalp roller with micronized needles plus an exclusive liposomal polypeptide serum to further enhance the results. The theory behind this treatment system is that by enhancing collagen production the micro-circulation within the scalp is increased which in turn creates new hair growth. MTS claims 100 percent results in creating new hair growth within the first three months of usage and also an 80 percent reduction in hair loss. This is truly a unique system but does carry a high price tag. One plus though is the scalp roller only has to be purchased once.

SOURCES FOR MTS HAIR RESTORATION COMPLEX

1. http://www.ebskin.com
2. http://www.microneedle.com/main/index.html

ADDITIONAL TREATMENTS GROUP N

NEW GENERATION HAIR CARE SYSTEMS

New Generation Hair Care Systems are marketed by California Pacific Research Incorporated that was founded by Bob Murphy. Most of the New Generation products are polysorbate based which is an ingredient that has been identified with halting hair loss and producing new hair growth. The original formula was derived from the research of Dr. Ilona Schreck-Purola of the University of Helsinki.

The formulations for both men and women include shampoos, scalp cleansers, an overnight formula, plus dietary supplements. Even though we consider the actual formulas based upon Dr. Purola's research to be excellent the quantity delivered with purchase is not cost-effective for long term treatment.

SOURCES FOR NEW GENERATION HAIR CARE SYSTEMS

1.   http://www.newgen2000.com

NISIM

The Nisim lineup for men and women includes shampoos and conditioners plus a specialized treatment. Utilizing an exclusive blend of all natural ingredients that reduce dihydrotestosterone they claim an 85% success rate when their products are employed on a regular basis. Some of the chief ingredients are glycine soja, panax ginseng, castanea sativa, arnica montana, hedera helix, and geranium maculatum. These products have a lengthy history in the marketplace. Nisim International also sells the Kalo hair removal system and Milagro nail strengthening system.

SOURCES FOR NISIM

1.   http://www.nisim.com

NOURAGE

Nourage is a proprietary food/vitamin supplement developed in Switzerland to stimulate hair growth. The theory behind the product was to create an all-natural food supplement that would mimic the

194

building blocks of hair, which is keratin. After many years of research the makers claim they were able to create a formula that could be readily assimilated by the body. Treatment with the supplements is only prescribed for the duration of your hair problems.

SOURCES FOR NOURAGE

1.   http://www.nourage.com

NOURKRIN

Nourkrin is a top selling hair loss product in the United Kingdom and Ireland that classifies itself as natural food supplement for the hair. The formulations contain a combination of protein from marine extracts, cartilage from deep-sea fish, and various minerals and vitamins. Amazingly one of the chief components of the formula is glucosamine. For those not familiar with this particular supplement it is often used in conjunction with chondroitin for the treatment of various forms of arthritis. The product lineup for both men and women includes the all-natural food supplement, shampoos, conditioners, and hair sprays. These products also can be used with any type of hair loss including androgenetic alopecia, alopecia areata, alopecia totalis, alopecia universalis, and telogen effluvium. There is also one additional product specifically for male thinning hair that contains fenugreek and omega 3 fatty acids as added ingredients. Many leading hair experts in Europe including world-renowned trichologist Doctor David Kingsley endorse Nourkrin.

SOURCES FOR NOURKRIN

1.   http://www.nourkrin.com
2.   http://www.boots.com

NUTRIFOLICA

Nutrifolica advertises itself as a one-step topical all-natural botanical treatment for hair loss. Some of its primary ingredients are saw palmetto, haberno extract, and alpha hydroxy. In each case these particular ingredients have a specific role in the formulation. The saw palmetto acts as a DHT inhibitor while the extracts of the haberno pepper stimulate hair regrowth. Meanwhile the alpha hydroxy cleanses the scalp of excess oil, dead skin calls, plus other debris that would clog the hair follicles. Other ingredients also found in the treatment are sage, nettles, lemongrass, rosemary, nettles, hops, aloe vera, ginger, horsetail, green tea, and wild cherry bark.

SOURCES FOR NUTRIFOLICA

1. http://www.nutrifolica.com
2. http://www.hairregrowthformen.com

ADDITIONAL TREATMENTS GROUP O

ORIGENERE

Origenere is another company that prides itself in the use of superior all natural ingredients, patented as OrganoNutrients™, to combat hair loss. These formulas contain no parabens, sodium lauryl sulphate (SLS), ammonium lauryl sulphates (ALS), hydroquinone, methyllisothiazolinone, methylchloroisothiazolinone, or any mercury based compounds. As we pointed out earlier ample research is now indicating that some of the older hair care ingredients do more harm with regard to thinning hair than good. Their product lineup for both sexes contains shampoos, conditioners, creams, tonics, and their all new TR-1 Trichological Revolution Super Hair Formula. Common ingredients in the shampoo and conditioner are fenugreek and hops which we fully endorse for dealing with hair loss. The TR-1 formula is more apothecary based.

SOURCES FOR ORIGENERE

1. http://www.onlyhairloss.com
2. http://www.origenere.com

ADDITIONAL TREATMENTS GROUP P-Q

POLARIS LABS NR-O7 HAIR GROWTH TREATMENT

Polaris Labs advertises NR-O7 as a breakthrough treatment for hair loss sufferers and in many respects it is with regards to treating a receding hairline. The product itself contains a smorgasbord of ingredients long established as hair loss preventatives and hair growth agents. Some of the ingredients are 5% minoxidil whose absorption is enhanced by a next-generation liposphere technology combined with apple polyphenols to facilitate restoration of frontal hairlines. The addition of saw palmetto, adenosine, biotin, azelaic acid, lysine, apigenin, and retinols to this formula makes this a truly remarkable product. Furthermore the alcohol content is reduced to counter scalp irritation. As we have stated before this is an excellent combination for treating frontal hair loss while reserving less expensive variations of minoxidil on the crown portion of the scalp.

SOURCES FOR POLARIS LABS NR-O7 HAIR GROWTH TREATMENT

1. **May still be available on various web sites.**
2. **http://www.polarisresearchlabs.com**

PRAVANA BIOJEN 9

The hair growth system for men and women from Pravana Naturaceuticals attacks the problem of hair loss in three distinct ways. First it attempts to control access DHT, secondly it helps promote scalp circulation, and thirdly it removes the excess sebum and other debris blocking the follicle. It does this by utilizing a group of nine natural botanicals known as its Programine-T Complex. Some of the listed ingredients are Apigenin which is a citrus flavonoid utilized to promote microcirculation in the scalp. Oleanolic acid which has DHT inhibiting properties. Plus cleansing agents such as Biotinyl tri-peptide and natural alpha hydroxy acids. The product line-up includes cleansers, conditioners, a scalp energizer, plus a Rejuvenator with a mega dose of the Programine-T Complex. Chiefly sold in better hair care salons it is a reasonably priced hair loss solution.

SOURCES FOR PRAVANA BIOJEN 9

1. **http://www.sleekhair.com**
2. **http://pravana.com**

PROCERIN

Procerin is marketed as an all-natural tablet and topical serum for the treatment of androgenetic alopecia in men. The product contains an array of DHT blockers. Used once daily the formulas contain a seventeen-ingredient array of saw palmetto, gotu kola, nettles, magnesium, zinc sulfate, eleuthero root, vitamin B-6, pumpkin seed, and muira puma root. The topical serum includes gamma linolenic acid, grape seed extract, azelaic acid, saw palmetto extract, avocado oil, and nettle extract.

SOURCES FOR PROCERIN

1.   http://www.procerin.com

PROVILLUS

Provillus is a supplement composed of vitamins, herbs, and minerals meant to arrest DHT the leading cause of hair loss. The chief ingredients are saw palmetto dispensed as a mega dose and a proprietary blend of lesser-known herbs. The women's formula does not contain saw palmetto and seems to be primarily composed of B-vitamins and a few herbs.

SOURCES FOR PROVILLUS

1.   http://www.provillus.com

ADDITIONAL TREATMENTS GROUP R

REGENEPURE

Regenepure is a group of scientifically formulated treatment shampoos designed for men and women with a thinning scalp. Containing some of the finest hair loss ingredients available the DR version is formulated with ketoconazole for dandruff problems where the NT version is formulated without it. Since ketoconazole has demonstrated its ability as a hair growth stimulant and hair loss retardant we fully endorse the use of it for everyone. Other noted natural ingredients are saw palmetto, Emu oil, caffeine, niacin, and zinc oxide. The treatments themselves offer a less costly alternative to the Revita line of products. As an added plus these shampoos are also non-hypoallergenic and contain no sulfates, harsh chemicals, or artificial ingredients.

SOURCES FOR REGENEPURE

1.   http://www.regenepure.com

REJUVE3

The Rejuve3 Hair Loss System is a product of Derjers International. It is advertised as a powerful hair cleansing system to rejuvenate the scalp. The product line-up includes a renewing scalp cleanser, repairing shampoo, and a revitalizing conditioner. The predominant ingredient in the formulas seems to be Polysorbate 80.

SOURCES FOR REJUVE3

1.   http://www.derjers.com

REMINEX

Reminex offers an all-natural alternative for gray hair as compared to messy creams and lotions that must be used regularly to eliminate the root problem. This proprietary vitamin and herbal formula even offers a full money back guarantee if you are unsatisfied with your results. The product line-up now includes a shampoo with similar ingredients as the supplement and is helpful in eliminating the brassy overtones common to gray hair.

SOURCES FOR REMINEX

1.   http://reminex.com

REMOX

Doctor Oscar Klein first developed the Remox brand. The initial formula combined the benefits of minoxidil (5%) with tretinoin. This combination is considered one of the more potent formulations in fighting male and female hair loss. Now there are versions of Remox containing spironolactone, azelaic acid, progesterone, and finasteride all powerful hair growth agents. The product lineup includes shampoos, gels, sprays, foams, lotions, and vitamin supplements.

SOURCES FOR REMOX

1.   http://www.physicianshairgrowth.com

RENAXIL (L'OREAL)

Renaxil is a product from the world renowned L'Oreal of Paris. Marketed as a cure for thinning hair its primary ingredients are aminexil and medecassoside. The former a known hair growth agent developed by L'Oreal and the latter a hair loss retardant. The formula also contains advanced polymers that give added thickness to the present hair. The treatments predominantly for men are sold in a light and advanced offerings based upon the degree of hair thinning. Usage is required twice a day for six weeks and then a maintenance phase of two to three times a week thereafter. Purchasing of these particular treatments seems confined to Europe and Australia but can be found in the United States. Based upon the short duration to obtain results, pricing, claimed results, guarantee, and company reputation the cost seems reasonable. According to the accompanying literature you should obtain noticeable results within six weeks.

SOURCES FOR RENAXIL (L'OREAL)

1.   http://www.ozhairandbeauty.com

RETANE

Nutrica Retane is an all-natural botanical hair tonic scientifically formulated to quickly stop hair loss in men and women, help promote new hair growth, and ensure optimal hair and scalp health. It is a one-product lineup that can be utilized by both males and females with regimes based upon the severity of the hair loss. Ingredients found in the formula are inositol, biotin, vitamin B5, folic acid, protodioscin, vitamin E, aloe vera, and ginseng panax extract. Scientific research conducted by Nutrica determined the formulation was able to halt hair shedding in eighty-six percent of patients within a four week period. This effect was observed with a variety of alopecia's especially the aerates.

SOURCES FOR RETANE

1.   http://www.retane.com

REVALID

Revalid offers a Swiss company offers a complete line of hair loss products for men and women. The makers claim they have the panacea for thinning with hair their patented ingredient Biobranil. The product of note here is their tonic energizer which contains caffeine. As you might know that particular drug has been identified as possible cure for baldness and as a hair loss preventative. The full line-up of products contains a shampoo, conditioner, cream, balm, and vitamins. Somewhat pricey in the US bargains can be found at such places as E-Bay.

SOURCES FOR REVALID

1. **http://www.revalid.net**

REVIVOGEN

Revivogen is marketed by Advanced Skin and Hair Incorporated as an all-natural dermatological tested solution for hair loss and thinning hair. Its formulations for both men and women include a targeted therapy plus shampoos and conditioners for hair loss. The composition of the products includes known DHT blockers effective in reducing both types 1 and 2 five alpha reductase. As mentioned in our prior work these two factors are largely responsible for most people's hair loss.

The active ingredients include gamma linolenic acid, alpha linolenic acid, linoleic acid, oleic acid, azaleic acid, vitamin B6, zinc, saw palmetto extract, beta sitosterol, and procyanidin oligomers.

SOURCES FOR REVIVOGEN

1. **http://www.revivogen.com**

REVLON INTERACTIVES

Without a doubt one of the largest hair care manufacturers in the world isn't going to be without a lineup of fine hair loss products. In this case Revlon's Interactives offers women a full regime of shampoos, conditioners, tonics, and unique patch delivery system for your thinning hair. This patch known as Intragen 5 was developed with the idea in mind that there is no one unique factor that causes female hair loss therefore it reacts to multiple conditions. These particular factors being related to the genetics, seasonal changes, stress, health, and hormonal changes women may be experiencing. Revlon claims an 80 percent success rate with its Interactives system which is predominantly found in Europe and the UK.

Intragen 5 largely accomplishes it mission through:

1. Naturally blocking hormonal agents responsible for female hair loss.
2. Protecting capillary cells from premature aging.
3. Stimulating oxygenation and cellular nutrition.
4. Increasing the production of new cells.
5. Reducing excess sebum in the scalp.

SOURCES FOR REVLON INTERACTIVES

1. **http://patchantichute.com**

ADDITIONAL TREATMENTS GROUP S

SAINI HERBAL SCALP AND HAIR CONDITIONER

Saini Herbal is marketed by Positive Trends Incorporated as all herbal formula derived from inhabitants of the northern parts of India. Composed of plant extracts the formula is advertised as both a deep cleanser for the scalp and hair rejuvenator. Some of the listed ingredients are bhringaraj, amla, shikakai, camphor, and rasult. This product for both men and women is also sold as a dandruff remedy.

SOURCES FOR SAINI HERBAL SCALP AND HAIR CONDITIONER

1. **http://www.sainiherb.com**

SAMSON'S SECRET

This product is named after the legendary biblical character Samson who drew his tremendous strength from his long tresses of hair. This all-natural botanical formula contains a blend of herbs to be applied topically to encourage optimal hair growth and increase the strength and beauty of the present hair. The chief ingredients are burdock, cayenne, rosemary, sage, oat straw, sarsaparilla, nettle, spirulina, and kelp. Most of these are known DHT blockers and hair growth stimulants.

SOURCES FOR SAMSON'S SECRET

1.   http://www.samsonssecret.com

SCALP MED

Scalp Med has become particularly well known through television advertising and array of infomercials. The main ingredient in Scalp Med is the same as Rogaine, which is minoxidil. The makers of Scalp med say that their product contains extra ingredients, which make their formula more effective, less greasy, and less irritating as compared to the competition. What those particular ingredients are though is not known. The product formulations are for both and men and women. The lineup of products includes the primary growth treatment Vitadil and Nutrisol which contains and array of vitamins, minerals, herbs, and amino acids. Plus the cortex enlarger or thickening spray. Additional add-ons are the Detoxifying Cleanser system and a mega multi-vitamin formula.

SOURCES FOR SCALP MED

1.   http://www.scalpmed.com

SEGALS SOLUTIONS

Segals Hair Loss Solutions had its birthplace in South Africa when the founder of the company noticed a particular tribe had much healthier heads of hair than other tribes he had observed. Procuring the information from the natives, as to the reason why, he set about creating a similar compound for enhancing hair growth. Thus was born Segals Hair Loss Solutions. These all-natural formulations for both men and women include shampoos, conditioners, and the special root stimulator, which has been passed down through the Segal family since 1970. Segal claims the formulas reduce sebum buildup that clogs the hair pores, increase blood circulation within the scalp, and enhance the appearance and condition of the hair. Even though Segal claims many of the formulations are family secrets they do seem to utilize some known well-known hair loss ingredients such as polysorbate 80, biotin, and saw palmetto.

SOURCES FOR SEGALS SOLUTIONS

1. http://www.segalshaircare.com

SEPHREN

Sephren is a product specifically formulated for women experiencing hair loss. The theory behind this product is many situations such as childbirth, menopause, birth control, and thyroid conditions can cause hormonal imbalances in females so a unique formula is required to combat their hair loss. Voila, you have Sephren, which includes a vitamin supplement and a scalp serum for combating thinning hair. Ingredients included in the supplement are vitamin B-6, biotin, magnesium, horsetail silica, and para-amino benzoic acid (PABA). Ingredients included in the topical serum are jojoba oil, grape seed oil, cedarwood oil, thyme oil, rosemary oil, and lavender oils. This particular combination of oils is well known in aromatherapy for its hair growing properties.

SOURCES FOR SEPHREN

1. http://www.sephren.com

SESKAVEL

Seskavel offers an interesting take on combating hair loss by utilizing sophora root, sabal, and 5 alpha avocuta. Sophora root has been associated with stimulating the anagen phase of hair growth while at the same time combating the demodex mite. Sabal extract on the other hand has DHT inhibiting and anti-bacterial qualities. Finally 5 alpha avocuta is excellent in combating seborrhea and stimulating the scalp's circulation. The product line-up for men and women includes a shampoo, lotion, and dietary supplement. Some of the other ingredients included in the formulas are saw palmetto, Taurine, soy, and oatmeal. Again this is another group of products without wide-spread distribution except in the United Kingdom.

SOURCES FOR SESKAVEL

1. http://www.sesdermausa.com

SIGMA SKIN HAIR REGROWTH SYSTEM

The Sigma Skin Hair Regrowth System is another breakthrough group of products from DA Laboratories. The formulations are meant for people suffering from pattern baldness that has significantly affected both the frontal hairline and crown portions of the scalp. Included in the system are hair growth shampoos, a minoxidil 5% spray solution, and a leave in hair conditioner. When combined the products work synergistically to cure both bald spots and hair recession in the frontal portions of the scalp.

What's truly unique about these products is they are the first to utilize apple polyphenols. Japanese research has long maintained that these particular polyphenols from apples can be a cure for male and female pattern baldness. Other included ingredients are adenosine, caffeine, retinols, and biotin. Bottom line is this is not an inexpensive solution but more for the man or woman who has everything. In regard to the minoxidil spray you can substitute a cheaper brand and only use parts one and three of the system.

SOURCES FOR SIGMA SKIN HAIR REGROWTH SYSTEM

1. http://www.sigmaskin.com

SMART ORGANIC PRODUCTS

Smart Organic Products are receiving a heavy advertising push with claims they have the ideal products for male and female hair loss. The lineup includes a shampoo, conditioner, and scalp serum. Their chief claim to fame is that the formulas contain Rooibos. Other listed ingredients are apple polyphenols and green tea.

At ThinScalp.com and ThinningScalp.com we were some of the first to report on the use of Rooibos, apple polyphenols, and green tea as baldness preventatives and hair growth agents.

SOURCES FOR SMART ORGANIC PRODUCTS

1. http://www.smartorganicproducts.com

SPECTRAL DNC, RS, L, N, S

Spectral DNC had its birth in Europe largely because of stiff US laws regarding the recombination of pharmaceutical agents. It advertises itself as the "world's most effective topical hair loss treatment". It is now approved for sale in the United States. The original formula was chiefly composed of 5% minoxidil plus retinol and aminexil. The latter being a hair growth stimulator developed by L'Oreal of Paris. Spectral DNC sets itself apart from other hair loss formulas with its microscopic nanosome delivery system that allows for deeper penetration into the skin. The newer formulation includes adenosine and procyanidins of B-2 and C-1. This is definitely one of the more potent recombinations of minoxidil and caution should be observed if you have known problems with this ingredient.

The Spectral array of products also includes the RC and DNC-L lineup. The RC formulation is minoxidil free where the DNC-L formula is marketed as a cream for the most difficult cases of alopecia.

SOURCES FOR SPECTRAL DNC, RS, L, N, S

1.   http://www.folica.com
2.   http://www.spectraldncs.com

ADDITIONAL TREATMENTS GROUP T

TELOSTATIN

Telostatin Hair Restoration Gel claims to be the only product currently produced that stimulates the anagen phase of hair growth while at the same time suppressing the catagenic (resting) and telogenic (loss) phase of the human hair growth cycle. It does so by adding a specific bioactive polypeptide - Target Activator 5 (TA$_5$) to its compound. Other ingredients included in this formulation were added to control seborrhea and the parasites common to Demodex. By controlling these maladies supposedly blood flow is increased within the scalp. Activor, the makers of this product, feels that this enhanced blood circulation is an integral part of increasing hair growth and reversing pattern baldness. Nioxin in some respects followed a similar approach with Semodex but lacked the growth ingredients found in this product. Telostatin Hair Restoration Gel is not widely distributed and carries a hefty price tag.

SOURCES FOR TELOSTATIN

1.   http://www.herbalremedies.com

THOMAS LABORATORIES

Thomas Laboratories is a company of long standing in the hair loss community selling a proprietary group of products for both men and women to combat excessive hair loss. The products are further individualized to the condition of the hair and the degree of hair loss the client is experiencing. The product lineup includes their exclusive Formula 88 Scalp Cleanser, Formula TX Scalp Accelerator, Namron Plus Multivitamin-Mineral Complex, and a protein shampoo. The company was founded by Doctor Paul A. Thomas and touts an existence of 75 years.

SOURCES FOR THOMAS LABORATORIES' PRODUCTS

1.   http://www.thomaslaboratories.com

THYMUSKIN

Thymuskin was originally developed as a cancer treatment in Germany. Researchers soon discovered when the ingredients were applied topically it induced hair growth and halted hair loss. The theory behind the products is pattern baldness is the result of an auto-immune disease. As a result of this, as pointed out in product literature, the body regards the hair follicles as something growing too fast therefore it sends out white blood cells (leukocytes) to attack the hair follicles, which it considers to be foreign invaders. The hair follicles become so damaged by the attack of the leukocytes that they let go of the hair strands, and hair falls out. Eventually, the result is pattern baldness.

The primary ingredient was originally thymus extract derived from young calves but this has changed with evolvement of the product line. Now a synthetic thymus extract is utilized. Thymuskin advertises that most cases of pattern alopecia can remedied with nine to twelve months.

SOURCES FOR THYMUSKIN

1. **http://www.thymuskin.com**
2. **http://www.thymuskinshampoo.com**

ADDITIONAL TREATMENTS GROUP U-V

VIVISCAL

Viviscal is a proprietary product developed in Finland. The key ingredients are marine extracts sold as a food supplement. Viviscal is advertised as working through the bloodstream providing the body with correct balance of needed nutrients thus nourishing the hair follicle. The product has a loyal following and along with strengthening and thickening one's current hair it also has beneficial effects on the skin and nails.

The product lineup, for both men and women, includes hair shampoos and conditioners, a scalp lotion, and the extract tablets. Viviscal is now owned by the makers of Nourkrin which is another well-known hair loss product chiefly marketed in the United Kingdom.

SOURCES FOR VIVISCAL

1. **http://www.viviscal.com**

ADDITIONAL TREATMENTS GROUP W-X-Y-Z

X5 HAIR LASER

The X5 Hair Laser is one of the latest innovations from Spencer Forrest the makers of another well-known hair loss product, Toppik. Spencer Forrest claims this is the most powerful hand-held laser on the planet for treating hair loss. Operating at 60 milliwatts at precisely 650 nanometers the creators of this product argue that this is the ideal frequency for creating hair growth plus it's comparable to clinical lasers costing as much as fifty thousand dollars. What's truly unique about this device though, including its dimensions, is a patent pending design that conforms to the curvatures of the scalp. By doing so the X5 is able to create greater penetration free of the effects of scalp hair. Some of the advantages of this device that can be utilized by both men and women are:

1. A onetime expense with a two-year warranty.
2. No harmful side effects associated with internally consumed agents.
3. A three times a week schedule of use should deliver results.

SOURCES FOR X5 HAIR LASER

1.   http://x5hairlaser.com

ZINCPLEX SCALP CARE

Scalp Health makes the claim that their products are the number one natural solution for numerous scalp problems including thinning hair. The primary ingredient in their products is a patented formulation of Zinc PCA. According to Scalp Health zinc plays an essential role in the proper functioning of the hair and skin and readily point out the fact that 22% of the body's zinc supply can be found in the scalp. In other words when the body experiences a short supply of this essential mineral it develops maladies such as itchy dry scalp, seborrhea, sebum plugs, hair loss, scalp acne, oily hair, funguses, and dandruff. In essence zinc acts as a DHT blocker, scalp purifier, infection fighter, bacteria killer, and scalp oil regulator. Hence with proper zinc supplementation many of these problems can be alleviated.

The product line-up includes shampoos and conditioners. Other ingredients included in the formulas are tea tree oil, aloe vera, thyme, sage, fenugreek, burdock, and biotin.

SOURCES FOR ZINCPLEX SCALP CARE

1.   http://www.scalp-health.com

QUICK LINKS TO ADDITIONAL HAIR LOSS SITES

1. Adenogen http://www.evecare.com
2. Advecia http://www.progressivehealth.com
3. American Crew Trichology Hair System http://americancrew.com
4. Aminexil http://www.antiaging-systems.com
5. Aminexil http://www.hairloss-hair-loss.com
6. Ancient Secrets http://www.make-hair-grow-faster-7pe.com
7. Arcon Tisane http://www.arcon-international.de
8. Avacor http://www.avacor.com
9. Biofen http://www.biofen.com
10. Bioscal and Bioscalin http://www.hairgrowthpartner.com
11. Cellex-C Hair Recovery Complex http://www.cellex-cjunior.com
12. Clair's http://www.clairshairtreatment.com
13. Corvinex http://www.corvinex.com
14. Cre-C Shampoo http://www.justbeautysupplies.com
15. Crinagen http://www.raztec.com
16. Curetage http://www.curetage.com
17. Dead Sea http://deadseaserum.com
18. Dermendox http://www.folica.com
19. Dr. Lewenberg http://www.baldspot.com
20. Eucapil http://www.eucapil.com
21. Exo Balance http://www.exobalance.com
22. Fabao http://www.fabao.com
23. Ferm-T Super Hair Energizer http://www.superhairenergizer.net
24. FNS Osmotics http://www.osmotics.com
25. Hair Cubed http://www.haircubed.com
26. Hair Genesis http://www.hairgenesis.net
27. Hair Growth Laser http://www.50lasers.com
28. Hair Prime http://www.unibio.com
29. Hair Signals http://www.onlyhairloss.com
30. Hair Stimulator http://shop.hlpcproducts.com
31. Hair-Tek http://www.hair-tek.com
32. Har Vokse http://www.harvokse.com
33. Herbal Essentials http://www.endhairlossnaturally.com
34. Herbal H http://www.herbal-h.com
35. HLLC Scripts http://www.wheredidmyhairgo.com

QUICK LINKS TO ADDITIONAL
HAIR LOSS SITES 2 CONTINUED

36. Inneov Hair Mass http://www.parafarmacia-online.com
37. Just Natural http://www.justnaturalskincare.com
38. Juveline http://www.elsomresearch.com
39. Keracyte b http://www.keracyte.com
40. Keratase Densifique Large Internet Resellers
41. Kerium http://www.pharmamundi.com
42. Kevis http://www.kevis.com
43. Korres Anti-Hair Loss Shampoo
    http://www.lookfantastic.com
44. Lacinia http://www.lacinia.com
45. Lanadil http://www.bebeautiful.com
46. Laser Comb http://www.hairmax.com
47. Leonor Greyl http://www.beautybridge.com
48. Melancor http://www.melancor.com
49. Minoxidil Max http://www.solutions4hairloss.com
50. MTS Hair Restoration Complex http://www.ebskin.com
51. New Generation http://www.newgen2000.com
52. Nisim http://www.nisim.com
53. Nourage http://www.nourage.com
54. Nourkrin http://www.nourkrin.com
55. Nutrifolica http://www.nutrifolica.com
56. Origenere http://www.origenere.com
57. Polaris Labs NR-07 http://www.polarisresearchlabs.com
58. Pravana Biojen 9 http://www.sleekhair.com
59. Procerin http://www.procerin.com
60. Provillus http://www.provillus.com
61. Regenepure http://www.regenepure.com
62. Rejuve3 http://www.derjers.com
63. Reminex http://reminex.com
64. Remox http://www.physicianshairgrowth.com
65. Renaxil http://www.ozhairandbeauty.com
66. Retane http://www.retane.com
67. Revalid http://www.revalid.net
68. Revivogen http://www.revivogen.com
69. Revlon Intcractives http://www.hairsupermarket.com
70. Saini Herbal http://www.sainiherb.com
71. Samson's Secret http://www.samsonssecret.com
72. Scalp Med http://www.scalpmed.com
73. Segals Solutions http://www.segalshaircare.com

QUICK LINKS TO ADDITIONAL
HAIR LOSS SITES 3 CONTINUED

74. Sephren http://www.sephren.com
75. Seskavel http://www.sesdermausa.com
76. Sigma Skin Hair Regrowth System
    http://www.sigmaskin.com
77. Smart Organic Products
    http://www.smartorganicproducts.com
78. Spectral DNC http://www.spectraldncs.com
79. Telostatin http://www.herbalremedies.com
80. Thomas Laboratories
    http://www.thomaslaboratories.com
81. Thymuskin http://www.thymuskin.com
82. Thymuskin http://www.thymuskinshampoo.com
83. Viviscal http://www.viviscal.com
84. Viviscal http://www.viviscal.co.uk
85. X5 Hair Laser http://x5hairlaser.com
86. ZincPlex http://www.scalp-health.com

DISTRIBUTORS FOR A VARIETY
OF HAIR LOSS PRODUCTS

1. http://www.haircountry.com
2. http://www.sn2000.com
3. http://www.folica.com
4. http://www.minoxidilshop.com
5. http://www.hairlosswatch.com
6. http://www.hair1.com
7. http://www.baushbees.com
8. http://www.wheredidmyhairgo.com

ABBREVIATED DIRECTORY

PRODUCT DIRECTORY

<u>NOTES</u>

www.ingramcontent.com/pod-product-compliance
Lightning Source LLC
Chambersburg PA
CBHW050115280326
41933CB00010B/1104